The 5:2 Diet

Feast for 5 Days
Fast for 2 Days
to Lose Weight and
Revitalize Your Health

KATE HARRISON

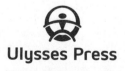

Ulysses Press

Published by
Ulysses Press
P.O. Box 3440
Berkeley, CA 94703
www.ulyssespress.com

ISBN: 978-1-61243-269-4
Library of Congress Catalog Number 2013942631

Printed in the United States by Bang Printing

10 9 8 7 6 5 4 3 2 1

Acquisitions Editor: Katherine Furman
Managing Editor: Claire Chun
Editor: Lauren Harrison
Proofreader: Elyce Berrigan-Dunlop
Indexer: Sayre Van Young
Cover design: Double R Design
Interior design: Jake Flaherty

Distributed by Publishers Group West

IMPORTANT NOTE TO READERS

Contents

A Letter from the Author

June, 2013

Dear Reader,

Ten months ago, I watched a TV program that changed my life. I almost didn't write that line, because it sounds so cheesy, but it happens to be true. Sixty minutes of viewing set the scene for a huge change in my attitude toward dieting, introduced me to an exciting new branch of medical science—and gave me the tools to begin transforming my body.

Of course, I've had to do the hard work myself, but the program opened the door to the world of intermittent fasting and calorie restriction, the official name for an approach to health and diet that is gaining huge numbers of followers around the world. What began with a science show on British TV—inspired by some incredible work in U.S. universities and hospitals—has turned into a movement that is spreading to all corners of the globe. By autumn of last year, so many of my friends were trying it that I set up a group for us on Facebook. By January, it was the most talked-about diet in the UK, and before long the word of mouth successes were making waves in the U.S. too. My little Facebook group now has over 6,000 members from across the States, Australia, Europe, and Asia.

Many of those members shared their experiences for this book—experiences that are likely to inspire you to follow their lead!

What I've learned has made me feel in control of food, not the other way around. It's given me new hope that I can do something constructive to reduce my chances of developing cancer, dementia, and diabetes, which have had devastating effects on members of my family. It's a lifestyle I want to follow . . . well, for life.

The rapid popularity of this approach is typical of many hyped diets. You know the ones. They're flavor of the month, and then they drop out of fashion almost as quickly.

But intermittent fasting is one diet craze that is anything BUT crazy. It's sustainable, adaptable, and it might help you live longer. It's also very simple, and the "fasting" part isn't nearly as punishing as it sounds because—whisper it—you never have to go a day without eating. You simply work one, two, or more days of low-calorie eating into your weekly routine, and forget all about "dieting" the rest of the time. Until you step on the scale or try on the jeans that didn't fit two weeks ago . . .

And it's not just about how you look or how much you weigh—it's also about how your body works, right down to the cellular level. Reducing your calorie intake radically for short periods triggers changes in your body's metabolism and brain function that can cut the risk of the diseases we all fear: cancer, heart disease, Alzheimer's, and diabetes. There are benefits for your body and your brain as your body works hard to repair cells damaged by lifestyle and aging.

This "diet" is for people who don't diet. The health benefits are so great that people are choosing to adopt this approach to eating even if they don't have weight to lose—in my case, as I near my ideal weight, I have no intention of stopping. I'm going to carry on with the lifestyle because of the changes it's making. I have more energy than I have had in years, my outlook is more positive, and I feel—and look—younger.

The approach helps you to change your attitude toward food and eating for the better. In fact, many people prefer not to call it a diet at all, because so many calorie-controlled diets fail. It doesn't matter one bit whether you call this a diet, way of eating, approach, or lifestyle—what matters is that it's sustainable, sensible, and intuitive. And it works.

The benefits of fasting have been known in medical circles for some time, but finally this way of eating is going mainstream. There are no hidden gimmicks, no complications, no over-priced supplements or revolting meal replacements. In fact, this way of eating will save you money.

And it's definitely not just for girls . . . This is a diet that both men and women are adopting wholeheartedly because it's so flexible and fuss-free. Fast Days offer a "mini break" from worrying about food—and because you only have to stick to any kind of plan for a couple of days a week, you don't feel deprived. Plus, research suggests that even when given total freedom to eat what they like on Feast Days, dieters simply don't decide to binge or overcompensate. That's been true of my own experience and that of hundreds of others I know who are doing this—we adopt healthier habits without even thinking about it or noticing.

It's the ultimate practical guide to the most sustainable diet there is! *The 5:2 Diet* has all the information you need to start tomorrow. Or—if you're reading this before breakfast—you could even start today!

The book takes you step-by-step through embracing a lifestyle that suits your needs and goals. There is no proscriptive list of dos and don'ts, no list of "banned" or "sinful" foods. You work out the maximum number of calories you can eat on your Fast Days then stick to that limit for a couple of days a week, or once a week, or every other day—

it depends what suits you and how much weight, if any, you want to lose. Then you eat normally the rest of the time.

If it's that simple, why do I need a book about it? Well, maybe you don't—if you stick to 500 calories a day (if you're a woman) or 600 (if you're a man) on your "Fast" Days, then you'll almost certainly benefit. But, when I started following this regimen, I had lots of questions and uncertainties, and I looked in vain for a guide that would help me find the right approach. Which is why I've written this book.

Once I'd distilled all the information I could find for my own use, I decided it would make sense to put it together and create the consumer guide I couldn't find—so here it is.

It'll be your companion when you start, with lots of practical information, recipes, meal plans, and encouragement to help you launch this way of life and alter your body and approach to food for good. Pretty soon, this way of life should feel like second-nature, but the case studies and the remarkable scientific research underpinning this diet should help keep you on track. I've spoken to dozens of other 5:2 dieters, male and female, of all ages, who have shared their wisdom, success, and excitement about the changes they've seen.

I'm no doctor. I'm just a failed dieter who has found something that works for me, at last. And I am pretty certain it can work for you too. I happen to be a vegetarian and a baking TV show addict, but whether you're a dedicated foodie or not into cooking, a cuddly carnivore or a gluttonous veggie, a carb-lover or a party animal, you can make this fit your life.

Health Warning   I have no medical training, though I've always had a strong interest in food and nutrition. I'm going to share my experiences and those of other successful 5:2 dieters. But there are people who shouldn't follow this diet: children and teenagers, pregnant women, and people with compromised immunity. If you have type-2 diabetes, you should talk to your doctor as this diet could help but you need to do it under supervision.

In addition, anyone with a history of eating disorders should definitely not undertake this without talking to their doctor. In fact, even if you are otherwise healthy, talk to your GP—they're on your side, and if you are committed to losing weight, it'll make their job easier! It's also quite likely they'll know all about 5:2—many doctors are trying it for themselves!

This is the simplest, most grown-up diet in the world.   This diet—and this book—treats you like an adult. You pick and choose what makes sense to you. A lot of the science is new and evolving, so there are some questions that don't yet have definitive answers. My job is to offer you all the options so that, like me, you can find your own personalized way of working intermittent fasting into your life.

But have no doubt: this is working for me and thousands of others. Word on the diet has spread far and wide—because it works. And it could work for you too.

Of course, I love feeling slimmer, but this is about much more than vanity. Like most of us, I know that there are many diseases like cancer and diabetes that have blighted my family. Now at last I feel I can try something practical to improve my odds.

This book isn't about rules. It's about freedom. What's stopping you?

—*Kate Harrison*

Introduction: How This Book Works

The 5:2 Diet has three parts. **Part One** explains the thinking behind the diet, including medical and psychological research about why losing weight with this plan can boost your body in some incredible ways. These chapters are interspersed with my own diary, where I share highs and lows I encountered as I adapted to this new way of thinking about food and diet.

Part Two contains all the practical information you need to make 5:2, 4:3, 6:1, or Alternate Day Fasting (ADF) work for you. I've included information on how to prepare for the Fast Days and how to stay motivated, guidance on exercise and calorie counting, plus tons of real-life success stories and experiences to keep you on track.

Part Three focuses on food ideas for your Fast Days, with lots of simple options for meals and snacks to appeal to all tastes, including suggestions for seasonal eating and sample menus to stop you from feeling hungry. Finally, I know preparing food when you're on a diet can be a chore, so there are also ideas from 5:2 fans who've suggested their favorite ready-made meals. Many of us prefer to leave cooking till Feast Days when we're free to make the dishes we love! But there are also satisfying recipes should you want to make your food from scratch.

At the end, I've included a resources section for further reading, including chapter-by-chapter links to articles that offer more detail on relevant topics. I've abbreviated the links to make them easier to type into your browser if you want to find out more by going online. Alternatively, you can download a single list of links free via the 5:2 website: www.the5-2dietbook.com.

And the last item of all is the final installment of my diary, updated to include progress over the festive season and the new year. Spoiler alert! Keeping the weight off during family celebrations has proved easier than I ever expected. Are you ready to join the 5:2 revolution?

PART ONE
THE 5:2
REVOLUTION

What the Diet Does

How It Works

Why It's for You

Living the 5:2 Way— Feast, Fast, and Be Happy!

"I'm already on a diet. What makes this one different?"

Okay, I understand your skepticism. I've spent almost two-thirds of my life on a diet. And 99 percent of my adult life either dieting or feeling terrible about how I look. I'm not unusual. Most women I know—and increasing numbers of men—have a love/hate relationship with their bodies and with food.

OK, we can blame size-zero actresses for giving us unrealistic expectations about how we should look (and sending us to the cookie jar for comfort). Or we could pin it on multinational food companies or fast-food joints for trying to get us to eat more, more, MORE! But short of avoiding

Hollywood movies and growing all your food from scratch, there's little we can do about the external causes of what the press calls the "Obesity Epidemic."

What we can do is find a way of eating that works for us. And—to my astonishment—I think I might have done that at last, at the ripe old age of forty-four.

For me, and many others you'll hear from in this book, it's *revolutionary*.

What Life Is Like on 5:2

For breakfast this morning, I savored a chocolate and almond croissant from the best bakery I know, the one that's tormented me with its forbidden treats since I moved into a house approximately thirty-five steps from its doors. But it doesn't torture me anymore. Because thanks to the 5:2 Diet, I know I can indulge—even, occasionally, overindulge—but still lose weight.

Tomorrow I'll be fasting, one of two Fast Days a week (the 2 in 5:2), which are the only times I make a big change to how I eat. Strictly speaking, this isn't a true fast, because I can eat up to three small meals, but most 5:2 dieters do call these reduced-calorie days "Fast Days." I will eat roughly 25 percent of the calories my body actually needs. At that level, the way my metabolism works will change, but I won't feel faint or unbearably hungry as I probably would with a "true" fast.

I'll eat at lunch and dinnertime. In winter, I'll probably have soup for lunch, a vegetable curry side dish for dinner with some extra veggies, and perhaps yogurt or a piece of fruit for dessert. In summer, it's salads and fresh produce all the way. Yes, it is limited, but I don't care because the day after, I can forget counting calories and eat the things I enjoy.

Suddenly, food is not all about the "forbidden." I'm enjoying a balanced diet without feeling guilty about sharing a bottle of really delicious red wine or having a full Sunday brunch. So long as I keep a close eye on my eating habits for two days a week, I know I can enjoy a little of what I like the rest of the time and still lose weight.

Since I discovered this way of eating ten months ago, I've lost 26 pounds without cutting out any of the foods I love: cheese, chocolate, the occasional cocktail (make mine a mojito). I haven't gone crazy—I probably have shifted to a more balanced diet on my five "normal" days, but they haven't been conscious or planned changes. I simply have a much greater awareness of what my body needs and when it needs it. I eat when I'm hungry and without bingeing.

And I savor every mouthful.

But food is only part of the picture. I wake up with much more energy, my mood is positive even though I'm writing on a wet and cold day, and I feel relaxed but in control.

Don't Just Take My Word for It

I've surveyed dozens of dieters who are changing their lives for good. When Linda first contacted me in November 2012, she'd just fasted for the first time, having tried numerous diets over the years. She was planning to fast twice a week, and joked that if it worked, she'd be running marathons at the age of one hundred. Or at least, I thought she was joking. By January, she was definitely on track.

> I've lost 2 stone 4 pounds [32 pounds total]. I'm now 10 stone [140 pounds], so I wouldn't want to lose more than another 10 pounds. I've been doing 5:2 or 6:3 some weeks and I certainly aim on fasting one day a week for the rest of my life once I've lost the weight. I used to be really sluggish and generally had a nap in the afternoons (I'm 63 and retired) but now I've started the Couch to 5K running program (I'm on week two) and I aim at walking two miles each day on the days I'm not running. I've started running or walking rather than catching buses.   —Linda, 63

This works for all ages and both sexes. Software developer Andrew and his five coworkers all decided to begin the diet at the same time. Like many men, none had followed "named" diets before, but they were inspired by the simplicity and science of this approach. They've been tracking their progress for fourteen weeks now:

> I have lost 5kg [11 pounds] over 14 weeks, this seems to put me well within my target healthy weight. We have noticed how less tired we all feel and how the diet has become easy to do. In fact we look forward to our

diet days. Overall we have lost about the same but the point of the 5:2 diet is not really about losing weight, it's about health. The improvement in blood pressure, cholesterol, etc., is why we are doing it.   —Andrew, 42

Eleven pounds—an impressive loss. But how are they feeling about the diet? Thirty-four-year-old Sunil, a colleague of Andrew's, went in with a very clear target:

My main motivation is to reduce my cholesterol—I'm a British Indian, so [I] live mostly on an Indian diet, which isn't the best for reducing cholesterol. I wanted to try a diet that doesn't have a major impact on my life and this fits the bill. It's so easy. The first week or two are not hard, but it just takes a little discipline. I now don't even think about hunger on starving days. It feels normal. I find that my general appetite is less throughout the week—I used to have the urge to binge in evenings after dinner. I've lost 3.2 kilograms [7 pounds] and added an extra notch to my belt. I'm getting my cholesterol tested soon.   —Sunil, 34

Forty-one-year-old software engineer Kostas has always been athletic, but has still struggled with blood pressure and weight concerns. Until now.

I've lost 2 kilos [4.4 pounds], feel much better (psychologically), and less bloated, so I fit better in my clothes. The diet works, and there are hundreds of meals you can plan during a fasting day. The diet is keeping us healthier without depriving us of anything. Eventually, it will become a way of life. Now, even during my non-fasting days I am aware of what I eat and how much. I don't feel that I restrict myself from any kind of food that I like, because I can tell myself that I can eat it on my non-fasting days. My fasting days feel like I am cleansing myself.   —Kostas, 41

The freedom—and the cost savings—appeal to Myfanwy, who has lost 9 pounds. She was only slightly overweight to begin with and the loss has been steady. She's also showing a steady and welcome reduction in her blood pressure:

In terms of weight I am delighted to be slimmer and be able to wear things I never dreamed I would again. I can fit the diet around my life—work, teenage children, meals out, celebrations. It costs me nothing and saves me money (no lunches or snacks on fasting days). There's no complicated calorie balancing and no inevitable guilt when one cannot keep a diet up day after miserable day.   —Myfanwy, 49

The flexibility of the approach means people are trying out different variations. Several of the men I've surveyed have gone for a stricter fast, for simplicity and speed:

I have had limited success with restricted-calorie diets in the past, but was unable to keep up with them as a lifestyle. In under four weeks I've lost lots of weight

*and 2 inches off my waist. I love it! No calorie counting
makes it much more sustainable for me. I believe it's
much easier to stick to water and not eat on fasting
days than to consume the 500 to 600 calories that some
do.   —Rob, 42*

The Healthiest Diet?

So far, so good. We're losing weight and inches, and feeling
motivated. But there are other, even more important reasons why many of us have decided to do this diet:

*My mother had every illness under the sun, and I
don't want to follow in her footsteps. I have a young
family and wish to be around, plus the weight loss and
memory improvements would be a bonus. I've already
lost two stone [28 pounds] and inches from the stomach
(which would suggest a reduction in the risk of heart
disease). Plus, no saggy skin and my boobs have stayed
the same size, even though they're usually the first to
go on a diet!   —Fiona, 41*

*I wanted to lower my blood pressure and cholesterol,
and after two months, so far, so good. It's easy, and the
more you do it, the easier it gets. I like that it makes
scientific sense.   —Paul, 47*

*I'm doing this for weight loss and for health reasons.
My father has Alzheimer's, plus I have high blood
pressure.   —Sarah, 49*

Like Fiona and Sarah, I have concerns about my family's medical history, particularly diabetes and cancer. I'm still too young to be part of the official UK screening program, but I have mammograms every year because so many of my female relatives have developed cancer—including my mother, my aunt, and my grandmother.

But what I've learned since I began to research this diet has given me fresh hope. To give just one example: a major study has put women of my age with the same increased risk of breast cancer on a 5:2-style diet, and the results were very encouraging. The women have recorded good weight loss—which in itself helps to reduce the risk of developing various types of cancer. However, the researchers are also hoping that this kind of intermittent fasting might produce changes that work specifically to reduce the risk of breast cancer. The study highlights additional improvements in how the women's bodies respond to insulin—which also feels incredibly relevant to me as I am at very high risk of developing type-2 diabetes.

Whatever medical conditions your family is prone to, there's an excellent chance that 5:2 eating may be beneficial. This approach hits the jackpot because of the incredibly powerful effects it has on your body—and your brain.

The Diet That Succeeds Where Others Have Failed

The diet works very well for adults, but anecdotally, it seems it's proving especially popular among those thirty-five and over. It is around this age that we often begin to find it incredibly tough to shift our weight. We also become more aware of our own mortality and the health issues our parents or other family members are facing.

> *Couldn't fit in my clothes, saw my photos at my brother's fiftieth (awful), where we're all overweight, worried about joints, etc., scared of being disabled through fatness, felt that this offered an intelligent approach. Mum is losing her short-term memory and if fasting staves that off, I will give it a whirl. I need my brain. Feel a bit more hopeful of avoiding some of the health issues affecting my parents (and my grandparents before they passed away).* —Linda, 52

The Facebook group I set up (facebook.com/groups/the52diet—you're very welcome to join us) is full of motivating stories and wonderful "before and after" photographs from men and women of all ages and occupations—and they're reporting the same great results. Not just weight loss, but also improvements in a whole range of health issues and a powerful feeling that they're doing something positive for their bodies.

The 5:2 Diet has a huge advantage over other diets: it brings about physiological changes that help the body—and even the brain—heal itself.

Fasting does put stress on our systems, but the way we respond to that stress seems overwhelmingly positive. Research in humans and animals shows that fasting tends to lower the production of the hormone IGF-1, which plays a role in the development of cancer. Intermittent fasting activates processes that repair the body's cells and cuts insulin production, which in turn makes us less likely to lay down fat stores.

The effects on the brain are equally exciting. They include a potential reduction in the risk of Alzheimer's disease and other forms of dementia. On a more immediate basis, many people notice a lift in their mood, and fasting may even help with depression. These long-term medical effects are, of course, harder to measure on an individual basis than weight loss, but evidence increasingly suggests this way of eating has positive effects that far exceed the benefits of weight reduction alone. For more on the medical research and the science, see the "Fasting Recharge" chapter. The information is both fascinating and motivating.

Back in Control

There's another important benefit that wasn't featured in the television program that inspired me to take on this eating plan but has transformed the attitudes of many 5:2 dieters.

I'd more or less resigned myself to being fat and frumpy forever. I felt out of control, and very depressed about my lack of willpower, yet I couldn't seem to find a way to overcome that.

To my surprise, my Fast Days have had a profound effect on the way I think and behave, and not only when I'm restricting calories. The experience of reconnecting with my appetite, and relearning how to deal with occasional hunger pangs, has helped me and many other people get back in touch with how our bodies work.

I find fasting days very "cleansing." It has also made me realize that I can survive on a lot fewer calories than I thought I could. And periods of excess (e.g., vacations, Christmas, etc.) can be "put right" relatively effortlessly. —Claire, 43

Working really well for me. I like the discipline on two days (and the self-awareness of slight hunger discomfort), combined with complete freedom the rest of the week. —James, 43

I now believe very strongly that all those diets promising "you'll never feel hungry" have done us a disservice. Knowing the difference between eating because you need to and eating because you're bored/thirsty/fed up is a basic skill and one that can help you control and understand your weight issues. This way of eating has re-educated me about what my body needs—and when. Eating is less about habits and more about responding to my appetite, and I'm not the only one who feels this way.

> *It's bloody easy, and it's good to feel hungry. From years of dieting lore that advocated eating little and often, it feels like a relief to be able to skip meals and breakfast particularly.* —*Julia, 50*

In Chapter Four, I delve deeper into the psychology of this lifestyle change.

The Simplest Diet

The simplicity of this diet is what makes it so irresistible to many of us. You decide how many days a week to monitor calories, and then either do some simple math to work out your "limit" or go for the average of 500 for women and 600 for men.

Then you start. The foods you need on Fast Days can almost certainly be found in your cupboard, freezer, or definitely in your local supermarket. There's nothing specialized, no meal replacements, or exotic supplements to be bought at a huge expense.

> *I'm lazy when it comes to cooking so I keep things very simple: beans on toast for lunch and store-bought soup for dinner. I won't be winning* Masterchef, *but I don't care because keeping it fuss-free is really important in staying on this diet.* —*Katy, 30*

The only two tools that come in handy are a set of kitchen scales and either a calorie-counting book or access to the Internet so you can calculate your intake. But even those aren't compulsory. If you follow the ready-made food suggestions in Part Three of the book, you'll be able to do the diet without extra calorie counting.

> *I tend to stick to [frozen] chicken or beef dinners, or variations on that theme. They're all weighed out and have the calories on the boxes, so it saves weighing things and calculating calories.* —Sally, 49

I know pre-packaged meals aren't for everyone, but it's much easier now to find dishes that are low in preservatives and other additives—and someone else has done the portion control for you!

The Oldest Diet

Fasting is a part of almost all organized religions, suggesting that those faiths have long had an awareness of the benefits for mind and body in taking a break from eating or eating very simply and frugally. But you don't have to have any specific religious belief to follow the 5:2 Diet—what you're doing is taking advantage of ancient wisdom that is now being validated by cutting edge research.

Not for Everyone

As I said in the introduction, there are groups of people who should not make such major changes in eating patterns. This includes pregnant women or nursing mothers, children and teenagers, type-2 diabetics, and those with other chronic or acute medical conditions. If you have a great deal of weight to lose, 5:2 can work, but please do it under the supervision of your doctor.

This is also best avoided by people with a history of eating disorders or psychological issues around food or appearance. For most of us, eating less for a couple of days a week is easy to adopt, but like any habit, it can be taken to extremes that can damage your mental or physical health. If you have any worries, please, please talk to a specialist before considering the 5:2 or intermittent-fasting approach.

Indeed, to be safe, it's a good idea to talk to your doctor about this or any other dietary change. Sally is doing this already:

> *I'd suggest involving your doctor [or nurse practitioner] and going to be weighed there regularly too. That way they can keep an eye on you and a medical record of how the diet is affecting you. Most [offices] are set up to support weight loss. —Sally, 49*

I must admit I haven't gone down this route myself. I'd already been advised by my GP to lose weight and knew my basic health indicators—blood pressure, heart rate, fasting blood sugar—gave no particular cause for concern. But I did know I could count on their support to track the weight loss if need be. The last time I visited the doctor for a check-up, I was thrilled to show off my new weight loss, and the nurse wanted to know all about how I'd done it. Indeed, many health practitioners are reporting great results themselves.

In the next chapter, I'll be talking about the math of weight loss and how it relates to the 5:2 approach. But before that, with apologies to Bridget Jones, here's the first of my 5:2 diary entries, starting on the date that changed everything for me: August 6, 2012.

Kate's 5:2 Diary Part One

August 6, 2012

A Couch Potato Watches TV & Makes a Decision
Weight 161 Pounds
Mood: Guilty, Resigned

Today I am the fattest I've ever been.

Even though I've started three diets this year alone, I keep getting bigger. I weigh eleven and a half stone [161 pounds]—and am only five foot four inches tall (when I stand up *very* straight). So that gives me a BMI of 27.6—and anything 25 or above is overweight. Eleven stone [154 pounds] was bad enough—I thought that would be my mental limit, the moment where I took action, yet the weight is still creeping on.

My size 14 jeans [U.S. size 10] (which I always tend to think of as a 16 [U.S. size 12], as they're quite generously cut) are slicing into my waist, my bra is too tight and there are lumps and bumps showing when I wear anything but the baggiest of tops. Worst of all, my belly is wobbly—I've always been curvy, with big hips and boobs, but my tummy is now catching up.

Has anyone seen my willpower?

This is the slippery slope. I feel out of control, frumpy, middle-aged, and very, very cross with myself. I don't want to be gaining half a stone [7 pounds] a year, wearing a size 18 or more before I'm fifty, feeling ashamed to go on the beach because I look like the fat lady on a seaside postcard.

Yet my willpower is diminishing with age too. A few years ago, I managed to get to my lowest adult weight—a sylphlike eight and a half stone [119 pounds]—thanks to low-carb dieting the vegetarian way. I felt good on it, wore skinny jeans for the first time, and really enjoyed eating lots of lovely cheese, Greek yogurt, nuts, berries, and so on. And yet…

And yet even as people congratulated me on my success, a tiny part of me knew it couldn't last. I love bread, cakes, and desserts. I have a huge recipe book collection and adore farmers' markets and nice restaurants, especially Indian or Italian places. Could I really turn my back on pasta, rice pilaf, and baked goodies for the rest of my life?

Plus, something didn't feel quite right about eating such a restricted diet: cutting out one food group seemed wrong. Sure enough, the weight crept back on. I tried low-carb dieting again this last month, but I couldn't convince myself it was something that would last. Because, frankly, it won't.

Fat and fearful…

This is not simply about vanity anymore. Both my parents have type-2 diabetes—the kind that starts in later life—and I've seen the complications it causes to vision, joints, and the skin. Their diagnoses also mean my chances of getting it are very high.

Plus, there's the strong family history of breast cancer on Mum's side—and a friend who has recovered from breast cancer raised doubts about how reliant I was on dairy products on the low-carb veggie diet. Dairy is something she's minimized since she went into remission because she's concerned that too much of it might increase her cancer risk.

Though being overweight increases the risk of cancer too. It's hard to know what to do for the best.

How much more desperate do I need to become?

I've joined a gym again and am trying to go, but, realistically, three cross-trainer sessions a week are going to burn 1,200 calories maximum. Apparently to lose a pound of fat, you have to cut 3,500 calories from your diet, or do 3,500-worth of activity without eating any extra food. Gym-going alone is not going to be enough. I've joined a site, MyFitnessPal.com, to monitor what I'm eating, but it's labor-intensive and it doesn't include listings for the days I eat out, because it's impossible to know the calorie count of restaurant food.

Yesterday, I found myself Googling diet drugs—the kind that "bind" to the fat you eat and help you pass it before it gets digested. The side effects are utterly revolting and yet I went as far as filling in an online form to find out if I'd be eligible for them. I am, but apparently they're out of stock.

So I'm not alone in seeking a quick fix.

A lost cause...

Maybe I just have to accept this is the shape I'll stay. I could take down all the mirrors in the house to start with . . .

There's a TV program I'm going to watch tonight about fasting. The description of the show is intriguing. But let's face it—I don't have the willpower to do a "normal" diet, never mind a fast. I suspect it'll just give me even more to feel guilty about.

10:05 p.m.

Wow.

That was an amazing program . . . really fascinating, full of counterintuitive science and new information—plus fasting REALLY worked for the presenter.

Even better, it wasn't a "true" fast—he did still eat on his fasting days, just an awful lot less.

The potential benefits also seem to go way beyond weight loss. There's a possibility that "intermittent calorie restriction"—a more accurate but less catchy description than fasting—could reduce the risk of breast cancer, diabetes, heart disease, and even Alzheimer's.

This is a diet that could offer more than weight loss alone.

But I have been here before, with low-carb, high-fiber, tum/bum/thigh. The fact is, miracle diets don't exist.

Or do they? Maybe this time I might be able to get slim—and stay slim.

The Math of Weight Loss—and Why Fasting Adds Up

Slim people don't just look better by the pool. They also live longer. Those *rats*.

It's the reason your doctor monitors your weight and calculates your BMI—Body Mass Index—when you have a checkup. The BMI is a simple calculation based on your height and weight. (Some would say too simple: we'll talk about that a little later).

Basically, if your BMI is over 25, or 23 for some ethnic groups, you're officially overweight. And if it's over 30, you're classified as obese: the higher the figure, the higher the statistical risk of disease.

You can either calculate it with the formula below or by using the chart provided on page 196 in the Appendix.

$$\text{BMI} = [(\text{weight in pounds}) / (\text{height in inches} \times \text{height in inches})] \times 703$$

So if you are 5 feet 4 inches and weigh 161 pounds, you first figure out your height in inches—in this case it would be 64 inches. Then you multiply that number by itself, so 64 x 64 = 4,096. Now you divide your weight by that number: 161 / 4,096 = .0393. Finally you multiply that by 703, and you get 27.6, and that's your BMI. As a measure, BMI isn't perfect. You may have heard about athletes who train for hours a day yet are considered "obese" by BMI standards because they have lean bodies with high muscle mass. BMI is also pretty hopeless for measuring children. Plus, the risk calculations are based on large-scale studies so it can't tell you much about your personal, specific risks, which depend on so many other factors: family history, genetics, lifestyle, environment.

Also, BMI isn't the only indicator of the effect excess weight may be having on your health. Your waist measurement is also a strong predictor of your likelihood of developing cardiovascular disease, because it indicates how much "visceral" fat you've accumulated around your vital organs. This distribution of weight is important: "pear" shaped people with larger hips and thighs tend to have lower risks than "apples" who store more fat around the belly. The more you have, the higher your chances of developing heart problems or type-2 diabetes. The current NHS (the UK's National Health Service) guideline is that you are at greater risk if your waist (measured around your belly button) is more than 37 inches if you're a man or 31.5 inches if you're a woman.

Research presented at the European Congress on Obesity in France in 2012 advises to fine-tune that even more by aiming to keep our waist measurements to less than half of our height. So, in my case, I am 64 inches tall, so my waist measurement should stay under 32 inches (it has fallen from 32 to 29.5 since I began the diet!). The researchers promoting this method looked at data from 300,000 people and found the ratio between the two measurements was more effective at predicting the risk of diabetes, strokes, and heart problems than the BMI.

Lies, Damned Lies, and Basic Truths?

Of course, these risks are calculated based on averages across a population as a whole, and we each hope we'll be the exception to the rule. But before you write off the BMI or the waist circumference guidelines, remember statistics don't *always* lie. For every chain-smoking Great Aunt Winifred who was the size of a horse and ate like one, and celebrated her 100th birthday with a bottle of gin for breakfast, there are millions of us whose diets are damaging our health.

Excess weight can increase our risk of developing a range of diseases and conditions including:

- High blood pressure
- Type-2 diabetes

- Coronary heart disease

- Strokes

- Gallbladder disease

- Cancer of the breast or colon

- Osteoarthritis

- Respiratory problems

Of course, you could hope you're going to be the exception that proves the rule. Or you can try to maintain a "healthy" weight to keep the statistics on your side.

Whatever your BMI, the truth is you probably don't need a figure to tell you you've put on too much weight. My guess is that if you're reading this book, then you, like me, want to reduce your risks of these life-shortening, or quality-of-life reducing, conditions (as well as look better by the pool).

But, as we all know, losing weight is easier said than done:

I was first taken to a [weight-loss center] at the age of eleven and have been dieting ever since, sometimes with success, sometimes not. I originally lost weight when I was 17 by starving. I would have 1 ounce of All Bran (dry) in the morning, an apple at lunchtime, and plain salad in the evening. I used to tell my mum I was having lunch at [school] so that I didn't have to eat in the evening. I did this for 2 years and got down to 8 stone [112 pounds] which is too

*thin for my 5 foot 7 inches! Once I started eating
normally again the weight piled on. In my mid
twenties I went to a [weight-loss center] and got to
within 7 pounds of my goal weight. Again, as soon
as I started eating normally the weight piled on!
Then Weight Watchers, Slimming World, Rosemary
Conley [diet and fitness club] classes! I've tried Atkins,
Paul McKenna, Scarsdale . . . far too many diets to
mention!   —Jeanny, 53*

*I've tried all sorts—from The Cabbage Soup diet,
Slim-Fast, and the Beyoncé diet to Weight Watchers.
The one that's worked best for long-term weight loss
was [Weight Watchers]. I've had two successes there,
though gradually the weight has gone back on. I'm
greedy, really, it's that simple.   —Sarah, 49*

Eating Too Much Makes You Fat, and Other Annoying Things Thin People Say

People who don't struggle with their weight often have a
maddening habit of stating the obvious. "Losing weight is
easy," they'll say. "Couldn't be simpler. Eat less, move more."

Or they might point out the basic math: that if you consume more food (or calories) than you burn off, you'll put
on weight, and if you do the opposite, then you'll lose it.

"Oh, if I feel a bit chubby," they might say, pinching the imaginary inch (more like a millimeter) around their waists, "I just hold off the chocolate for a couple of weeks and I'm back to normal."

Well, good for them! For many of us, it's a lot more complicated.

Don't Blame Yourself, Blame Biology

There is a whole range of reasons why we gain weight the way we do, and a lot of them are external. But one important internal factor is our biology: we are designed to take in as much energy as we can in the "good" times to help us survive in the leaner times.

It's only very recently that starvation has ceased to be a threat to most developed populations. Now, we have incredibly wide choices of foods available to us—including all the healthy, fresh, minimally processed foods that doctors and diet experts recommend.

So why do so many of us make such bad choices? Because our bodies still act as though we're living in caves—rather than centrally heated houses—and still work as though we have to hunt and gather our food—instead of hitting the supermarket or even ordering our groceries online. What that means is, we naturally crave high-energy foods even if we don't need them. Our bodies can't think ahead. All they can do is react to now. So when sweet and fatty foods are available, we're programmed to like the taste and texture and to eat as much as possible so we can lay down fat stores for a nutritional "rainy day."

For our ancestors that made perfect sense, because there were plenty of times when there was no food to be had, so they had to rely on the times when they could eat everything that was available, to store energy for survival. But now, even if the economy is suffering, we tend not to cut back on food. And we still crave the sweet, fatty stuff.

Some people do manage to strike a balance, and stay slim. However, increasing numbers of us are becoming overweight or obese. We need a new strategy to help cope with external factors like those glamorous air-brushed actresses, enticing new foods, and energetic marketing campaigns.

Turning Biology to Your Advantage

Fasting and 5:2 lets us go back to basics. I think of it as reintroducing some of the "rainy days" our ancestors were all too familiar with by providing less energy from food, but unlike our ancestors, I do it in a controlled way.

How the body responds is incredible, as we'll see in the chapter "Fasting Recharge." More and more experts are convinced this is what we are designed to do. And the mind adjusts well too. Fast Days are limited, and Feast Days allow us to enjoy food, including the dishes we love, without feeling guilty. You might expect to binge, but research shows people rarely do. And if you shed the guilt, you begin to eat like a thin person without even trying. Here's what Sally has to say about it:

> *I like the idea that no foods are sins. As a lifetime yo-yo dieter, I've found something that really works for me. It isn't too hard to fit it into my lifestyle as it's flexible, and if I can't fast one day for any particular reason (e.g., a social occasion) I don't feel that I've failed. I just start again the next day.* —Sally, 49

I'm the same: within a couple of weeks I no longer felt deprived, or guilty, or ruled by my emotional response to food. As I felt less guilty, I was much more in touch with eating what I needed and no more. Which meant weight loss became less about the psychology and more about the math.

Is 5:2 Just a Different Way of Eating Less?

On the simplest level, 5:2 (or 6:1 or 4:3 or ADF) appears to work the same way as every other diet: you lose weight because you consume less energy (food) than you're using. The weight loss comes because, overall, you're eating less.

It doesn't sound very exciting, though some of the other physical and mental effects really are, but, ultimately, it's the same with all diets. It is possible with fasting, as well as some other diets, that there's what's known as a *metabolic advantage*: that is, eating this particular way will generate more weight loss (or, more specifically, *fat* loss) than can be attributed to the reduction in calories. But further research is needed.

Until we have more data, calories count on all diets. Take low-carb dieting. There's lots of talk about ketosis, which is a state where the body begins to use fat molecules for energy because it's deprived of the easier-to-process sugars it has access to when we eat carbohydrates. Those behind various low-carb regimens say that ketosis is one of the key factors in the weight losses observed by followers: it is seen by some almost as a "magic" state.

However, many studies have shown that it's much more straightforward than that. Low-carb dieters are consuming fewer calories than they did before, simply because they've cut an entire food group out of their diet.

That's what happened to me when I did it. I ate less, without really thinking about it, because I had fewer choices. Yes, I could eat butter, which I love, but what was the point without crusty bread or a delicious hot baked potato? I didn't feel hungry, particularly, because protein tends to make you feel fuller, which is one advantage of a high-protein diet (there are potential disadvantages too, as we'll see elsewhere). Of course, low-carb diets are also often high in fat, which is another factor. All that fat made me feel a bit sick after a while and I didn't want to eat anything at all. Therefore, I was eating fewer calories, almost by default.

But as soon as I started reintroducing the breads and potatoes into my diet (we moved to Barcelona, Spain, where *pan con tomate* is served everywhere, and a potato-packed tortilla is the default vegetarian option), I was no more able to resist these high-calorie foods than I was before my low-carb diet.

I boomeranged right back to my previous weight. And then some. Among the slim young things of one of Europe's funkiest city, I felt like a terrible frump. Which made me eat more.

The more extreme diets—cabbage soup, maple syrup, grapefruit—cut your calorie intake by restricting your diet and also your social life. Would anybody want to live on grapefruits for the rest of their life? I think it would feel like a very, very long life.

And as for cabbage soup . . . let's not go there. The bottom line about most diets is that they take the pleasure out of food.

The Basic Dieting Equation

$$X \text{ (the energy your body needs to function)} - Y$$
$$(3{,}500 \text{ calories})$$
$$= Z \text{ (a weight loss of 1 pound)}$$

As you can tell, algebra has never been my strong point. But simple arithmetic I *can* do.

And it works like this. It's estimated that to lose a pound of weight, we need to have a "deficit" of 3,500 calories; the same figure applies to putting weight *on*. If we eat 3,500 more calories than we need—over any period of time—we will potentially weigh a pound more. That helps to explain why even eating one more cookie a day, for example, can lead to significant weight gain over a year. On the positive side, it means small changes to reduce our daily consumption, for example, cutting out sugar in hot drinks, can have impressive cumulative effects.

So, to become a pound lighter, you must eat 3,500 calories less than your body needs. (Throughout this book, when I refer to calories, I'm referring to what nutrition labels list as calories.) Eat 35,000 calories fewer and that's 10 pounds gone.

That's the theory. As with everything in the diet/nutrition world, it's not quite that simple. A calorie is a simple measure of energy, but it doesn't reflect the different ways the body processes calories from fat, carbohydrates, and protein, which can affect how we store excess calories. Another factor in how much weight we might lose is exercise. We're encouraged to exercise as part of a healthy living plan, but muscle mass is denser and heavier than fat.

For the sake of simplicity, let's work with the 3,500 as it gives us a baseline. Whatever the exact numbers, it's very clear that to lose weight we must create a deficit to make our bodies turn to our fat stores for energy. The question is, how do you achieve this deficit?

For my entire dieting life, I've assumed that you must diet all the time. And that's where it's become tricky, because it's so hard to deny ourselves the foods we're programmed to crave. It's even harder to keep to a regimen when all you can see ahead is more deprivation.

All This Time, There Has Been Another Way

The 5:2 Diet—and all other types of intermittent fasting and calorie restriction—offers a radically different, though surprisingly obvious, solution. If you reduce your calorie intake more drastically, but for a limited period, you'll lose the weight. Because you aren't denying yourself the pleasures of food—or the social aspects of eating—the whole time, you stand a much higher chance of staying on track. Plus, knowing the medical benefits motivates you still further. It's win-win.

> *My other half is a chef, and having smaller portions or calorie counting 7 days a week just ain't going to happen, but I can manage 2. To my mind the big benefit is the 5:2 is far easier to fit round family life, socializing, etc., as one doesn't have to worry about it for the vast proportion of the time.*   —*Sarah, 49*

Doing the Math

So let's look at it in purely numerical terms.

A moderately active, average-sized woman needs 1,800 to 2,000 calories per day to maintain her weight, while for men it's 2,300–2,500. This is known as the daily calorie requirement (there are instructions for calculating your own DCR in Part Two).

Let's use Ms. Average as an example for now.

2,000 (daily requirement) x 7 (days of the week)

= 14,000 (total calories needed to maintain weight)

Conventional Calorie-Controlled Diet

If you're overweight and want to lose a pound a week (which many doctors suggest as a "sustainable" weight loss), you'd have to lower your weekly intake by 3,500 calories. In other words, you'd consume a maximum of 10,500 in one week, or 1,500 calories per day. This is how you'd aim to achieve that on a traditional calorie-controlled diet, where you're eating the same every day.

1,500 calories per day x 7 days
= 10,500 calories per week

That's actually a higher allowance than many calorie-controlled diets, but it still means calorie counting every day for a very long period: with 15 pounds to lose, for example, you're talking about fifteen weeks of counting and deprivation. If you're looking to lose 50 pounds, you're potentially facing about a year of constantly obsessing over what you're eating. That's boring, anti-social, and a constant reminder that you're "different."

5:2 Diet

Let's compare it to 5:2: you're cutting the calories more drastically for just two days of the week (or three or one, depending on what suits you best). The rest of the time you eat normally.

2,000 calorie Feast Days x 5 days = 10,000 calories

+ 500 calorie Fast Days
(25% of daily energy needed to maintain current weight)

x 2 days = 1,000 calories

= 11,000 per week

In this example, you're eating 500 calories more than you would by calorie counting every day. This would potentially slow down weight loss slightly, though many dieters I've spoken to say that on Feast Days, they tend to naturally eat a little less, so I suspect it evens out.

But there's another crucial point about 5:2—you don't actually need to calorie count the rest of the time. You can eat what you feel like. Many people really can't believe this at first, but research has shown that ICR (intermittent calorie restriction) doesn't lead to bingeing. On average, ICR dieters eat between 95% and 125% of what they need, but even the higher figure isn't enough to cancel out the fast days.

I can fast because I know next day I can have chocolate AND wine if I so wish. Funnily enough, because I can, I don't binge. —*Myfanwy, 49*

My "problem" is that having eaten low calorie foods for most of my life it's hard to eat anything like "normal" calories on my Feasting Days, so [I] will often eat a couple of [cookies] or have a glass of wine to make up the calories! —*Linda, 63*

Of course, if you decide to fast more often than two days a week—every other day, for example (known as Alternate Day Fasting or ADF)—the calorie deficit increases. So fasting on Sunday, Tuesday, and Thursday looks like this:

2,000 calorie Feast Days x 4 days = 8,000 calories

+ 1,500 calorie Fast Days
(25% of daily energy needed to maintain current weight)

x 3 days = 1,500 calories

= 9,500 calories total for the week

Many people on ADF do stick to three Fast Days, but it's advisable that you don't fast more often than every other day. There's a risk that you'll get fed up with restricting so often and quit—what you're looking for is a sustainable lifestyle.

What Are the Fast Days Like?

I won't lie, they can take some getting used to at first. We're so used to eating before we get anywhere near experiencing hunger that it can be odd or even alarming to begin with when our appetite kicks in.

It's easy, and the more you do it, the easier it gets. Eat some protein on your restricted days, and give the regime at least a month before considering if it works for you or not. —Paul, 47

Even just 500 calories for women and 600 for men is enough to keep you from feeling unwell, especially if you choose your foods wisely: there's much more about what to eat in Part Three.

Plus, believe it or not, hunger isn't a huge deal. When was the last time you felt hungry and not just thirsty or bored? Allowing yourself to experience hunger—and to see how little food it takes to feel full again—is a huge help when you want to have more control over your appetite and your eating.

Finally, and crucially, *it's only one day at a time*. In contrast to the daily monotony of "normal" diets, with 5:2 you only have to limit yourself for a couple of days (and they're not consecutive). It's so much easier to say no to a cake or a glass of wine when you know you can have it tomorrow than it is when your diet feels like a very long punishment for being fat.

Weight Loss Is Only the Start

So the math makes sense, and most people find this diet far easier to stick to than conventional calorie-controlled regimens (see the links list for research backing this up). But 5:2 is about so much more than weight loss. The evidence that fasting brings physiological and mental changes is growing all the time. As we'll see in the "science part" in "The Fasting Recharge" chapter, the secret is in your cells and your genes.

But before that, find out how I did in the first week of *my* fasting experiment. . . .

🗒 *Kate's 5:2 Diary Part Two*

August 9, 2012

First Fast—of Many?
Mood: Excited, Apprehensive, Unsure

I'm taking the plunge. Fasting is the future . . . maybe.

My boyfriend is skeptical, and other friends (who haven't seen the program) are also dubious. One talked in dark tones about "starvation mode" where your body responds to cutting calories by slowing down all its systems to keep you alive: that could mean when you go back to eating normal amounts, you put even more weight on.

But from my research online, the jury's out about whether that mode even exists. And if it does, then fasting one day at a time means you're not at risk of a metabolic slowdown.

When in doubt, Google It...

As I am self-employed and work from home, my first response to pretty much all my daily decisions is to Google them. Seriously. It's not something I'm proud of. Recently I've asked the big G where to rent a holiday cottage, how to answer my brand-new but complicated mobile phone, and whether it's true that Marilyn Monroe was severely flatulent (apparently so). So it's inevitable that I'm doing the same with 5:2.

The TV show was fascinating, but I still have lots of questions: how many meals a day should I eat on the "Fast" Days—is it better to eat one or three? What should my calorie target be on those days? Can I really eat as much as I like on my unrestricted or "feed days"? Apart from eating slightly less, is the diet different for women?

I fully expected to find lots of sites dealing with this approach, but what's out there doesn't seem to be aimed at the layperson—I found either scientific papers or pretty intense body-building sites.

What I did read seems to back up the potential health benefits, though. Plus, having worked as a producer at BBC myself, I know how stringent the guidelines are for making any health claim on a program, so I am certain the ideas *Horizon* featured will be sound—so I'm giving it a whirl.

It all adds up

The first thing I have to do is work out roughly how many calories I need to maintain my current (over) weight.

I could use the average fast day limit of 500 calories. But I'm keen to know exactly where I stand, so I use the calculators on the MyFitnessPal website. It's a very neat site which, so far, has mainly helped me record exactly how much I'm eating—too much— and made me feel guilty about my weekly intake of cava (what I really need is an app that stops me from opening the bottle in the first place).

My first step is to work out my Basal Metabolic Rate (BMR). That's an estimate of how many calories I need just to get through the day. The calculator tells me it's 1,365 which is a terrifyingly low figure . . .

Then I realize that's based on just keeping all your body's systems going. So I must factor in my activity level using the Harris Benedict Formula— which sounds a bit like an episode of *Sherlock*. Because I do some light exercise, I multiply my BMR by 1.375, which gives me a more generous 1876.87.

That's my daily calorie requirement (DCR)—the calories I should eat to stay at my current weight. Except of course I've been putting it on. Goodness knows how many calories I've put away to get this big.

The third calculation is the most important—for my new regimen to actually count as a fast (and potentially bring me all the health benefits that scientists are researching) I divide my DCR by 4. This comes to a slightly scary 469.25—even lower than the averages of 500 for women and 600 for men that presenter Dr. Michael Mosley quoted on the program. (There's a full guide to calculating your DCR in Part Two.) I go to the fridge and start reading labels on ready meals, soups, fruit, and veggie packaging.

Yes, it's low. But it's also . . . possibly . . . doable.

How often?

My final decision is how often I'm going to calorie restrict. On Twitter, Dr. Mosley said he's cut down from 5:2 to 6:1 because he was losing so much weight. Or for fast weight loss, there's alternate day fasting, but I'm a bit daunted by that. Right now, I don't know how I'll cope with even a single day of eating less than 500 calories in total.

5:2 sounds like a good start. Now all I need to do is, well, start. . . .

Fast Day 1: August 9, 2012

I wake up and try to pretend it's a normal day. A normal day where I happen to limit myself to a quarter of what my body needs, energy wise, and probably about a sixth of what it normally gets!

I eat the same breakfast most days—a mix of Greek yogurt and raspberries that I got to like when I low-carbed. It keeps me from feeling hungry till lunchtime. Trouble is, my usual portion size would take up more than half my calorie requirement for the day. So with the help of my digital scales, I measure out a doll-sized breakfast. If you've never tried measuring out 25 grams of yogurt, it's a tiny quantity, approximately one-fifth of a small container. Not very much. I use a tiny bowl and savor all four teaspoonfuls.

I've bought a big bottle of sparkling water, as my main "treat"; also, I know as a diet veteran that staying hydrated is super-important. Looks like these are the only bubbles I'll be getting today . . .

As lunchtime approaches, my mood is not helped by a rejection letter from the Women's Institute where I'd auditioned to be one of the speakers on their official list. I'd given talks to them in the past, but at my audition, the 100-strong panel decided I wasn't up to it. Though they do say I had a clear speaking voice and a pleasant personality.

Hmm. Good thing they can't see my grumpy face now, as I stand in the kitchen with the letter in one hand, the other one hovering over the packet of cookies.

But no.

I am better than that! And pleasant too.

I make myself a calorie-free black coffee and try not to think about lunch.

The department of weights and measures

Weighing is a good displacement activity. That, and reading the labels on the back of ready-made meals because frankly I don't trust myself to cook right now with so few calories to play with. I found a butternut squash dish in Marks & Spencer with just 140 calories for half a pack. OK, I think it's meant as a side dish, but it's quite filling for lunch and also allows me to treat myself to five cherry tomatoes, some arugula leaves, and a teaspoon full of balsamic vinegar as a dressing.

And, to keep it simpler, I have the same for dinner. Why mess with a winning formula? Dessert is the same as breakfast. And the total: 463 calories! Three under, should have had a couple more arugula leaves . . .

Time for bed

How's it been? Well, I've got a slight headache and have felt more peckish than hungry. Portions are small but it's been easy because the man of the house is out with friends tonight, so I haven't had to cook or resist sharing some wine.

But mainly it's been easy because I know I can eat exactly what I want tomorrow. I go to bed early. My tummy is rumbling, but my conscience is clear, and I hope to dream of what I can eat for breakfast in just over twelve hours' time.

What I ate to the last gram:

BREAKFAST
Greek-Style Natural Yogurt, 25 g: 34 cals
Ground Almonds 4 g: 25 cals
Strawberries, Raw, 53 g: 17 cals

LUNCH

M & S Moroccan Butternut Wedges with Roast
Vegetables, ½ pack: 140 cals
Peppery Baby Leaf Arugula Salad, 20 g: 4 cals
Balsamic Vinegar of Modena, 5 ml: 5 cals
Cherry Tomatoes, 5 tomatoes: 15 cals

DINNER

M & S Moroccan Butternut Wedges with Roast
Vegetables, ½ pack: 140 cals
Cherry Tomatoes, 5 tomatoes: 15 cals
Generic Balsamic Vinegar, 0.25 Tbsp: 3 cals

SNACKS

Greek-Style Natural Yogurt, 19 g: 25 cals
Ground Almonds, 5 g: 31 cals
Strawberries, Raw, 39 g: 12 cals

TOTAL FOR DAY: 463 CALS

The Fasting Recharge—Make Your Body Work Better

Weight loss is only part of the attraction of 5:2. This is the first "diet" that appeals to people who aren't overweight but want to take advantage of the incredible health benefits that fasting offers.

Increasing numbers of studies on both humans and animals suggest that there are unique benefits to be gained from fasting or restricting your calorie intake quite severely, even if you only do it some of the time.

We are talking about short-term changes—more energy, lower blood pressure and harmful cholesterol readings, higher levels of concentration—as well as long-term effects that help prevent the diseases that can affect our lives profoundly.

No wonder the weight loss begins to seem like the least important benefit!

I have concerns over dementia as it runs in my family so this side effect was particularly appealing. —Kirsty, 38

I've always eaten carefully in terms of nutrition but I am doing this for its possible health benefits. Alzheimer's, cancer, heart disease, high cholesterol, are all threats at my age. My cholesterol was 7.6, I have had breast cancer, my mother, at 94, has very poor memory. —Ros, 69

Why Does This Work?

Common sense might suggest that depriving the body of nutrients would be damaging and, indeed, it does put the body under stress.

But it's the body's response to that stress that seems to hold the key to the health benefits—just as a stressful job can bring out the best in us and help us achieve more, or we push ourselves in the gym and end up feeling better for it—putting your body under stress in a controlled way, can encourage it to heal itself and trigger processes that protect and repair.

Time for the "Science Part": The Secret Is in the Cells

The science bit is short, and sweet, and if you want to understand why this diet might have such huge benefits, it's worth focusing on this part! I've found it very inspiring to discover what's going on when I fast. But if you're not in the mood for theory, feel free to leave reading this till later. Part Two is the practical part, and I want you to use, and abuse, the guide as it suits you. No rules, remember?

Still with me? Great. We're all made up of cells—approximately 100 trillion of them in total. Think of TV images of "test tube babies" and in vitro fertilization where you can see the cells doubling in number over and over again as the embryo develops. Our cells continue their hard work throughout our lives. There are approximately 200 different kinds, all with different functions, and they're being replaced at the rate of millions per second. Some cells are constantly replaced, though others can't be. Even those that do multiply rapidly can only do so a certain number of times. It's this ceiling that is responsible for aging; as the number of skin cells drops, for example, your skin becomes thinner.

As part of their life cycle, some cells will also self-destruct in a carefully controlled house-keeping process known as apoptosis—they'll even "tidy up" after themselves as they prepare to die so they don't leave behind anything that could damage other cells. I love the idea of cells doing a Girl Scout–style good turn for the body, even as they approach the bitter end.

Another important process is autophagy. Literally "self-eating," this process can lead to the death of a cell but may also help it to survive under stress by recycling amino acids and removing damaged parts of the cell. The two processes work together to keep the body running efficiently.

But sometimes the cell production and destruction process goes wrong. When too many cells are produced uncontrollably it causes tumors, and the kind that then invade neighboring tissues are malignant—in other words, cancerous. Damage to brain cells can cause Alzheimer's or other forms of dementia, because as the structure of brain cells is changed they may die or become tangled up, and the chemical messengers that pass information around the brain no longer work as efficiently.

The more I've read about the science, the more amazed I've become at how hard the body works to regulate and protect itself. But time still catches up with us in the end . . .

Living Causes Aging

The trouble with life is that the very process of living causes damage to the body. Cells are damaged by the processes involved in producing the energy we need to function. Our bodies break down food into glucose (the simplest form of sugar) to use as energy, but that breaking down also damages proteins in the body and causes many of the signs and symptoms of old age.

Oxygen is part of that process, but while the body is making the energy, it's also producing free radicals that attack your cells in a process known as oxidative stress. When we're younger, we can cope better with this by "mopping up" the free radicals before they do too much damage. But it catches up with us sooner or later.

Can Eating Less Slow This Down?

At the simplest level, if you produce less energy, then you're potentially also causing less damage. That's one of the fundamental issues at the heart of much anti-aging research. It's been demonstrated in animal studies, from fruit flies to worms, mice to dogs, that eating less, or less frequently, can prolong lives. The exact chemical and biological processes involved are being researched, but the studies have already led to many people choosing to eat less than their recommended calorie requirements all the time, not just to keep their weight down, but to increase their life spans.

As someone with a keen interest in diets and nutrition, I've read a lot about "calorie restrictors," people who typically eat only 70 to 80 percent of their recommended intake, though they take extra care to eat very nutritious foods. Many people end up with BMIs of 19, 18, or lower, and frequently show reduced blood pressure and cholesterol levels. One of the main movements is called Calorie

Restriction with Optimum Nutrition, which is why they're known as CRONIES.

However, what I had read and seen on TV about CRONIES had put me off. The guy featured in the fasting program seemed fairly typical in that his diet looked expensive and pretty wasteful; for example, he ate the skin of fruit but discarded the pulp. And though he was very healthy, living that way all the time didn't look much fun! Now it seems 5:2 and Alternate Day Fasting may offer the benefits of that CRONIE lifestyle, but in a much more practical and laidback form. Instead of having to watch calories obsessively all the time, we can do it in short, sharp bursts that encourage the body to activate all the protective and reparative processes that may help us live longer and better.

It's Not Just How Much You Eat, It's Also What You Eat

Different foodstuffs have different effects on the body. For example, we've already mentioned that producing glucose stimulates those damaging free radicals.

According to the *Horizon* show, protein in particular seems to turbocharge the cell production process. The scientist interviewed, Professor Valter Longo, compared our bodies to race cars, where protein is making the cars race faster—what Dr. Mosley called "go-go mode"—with no chance at all to retune or recharge. Driving at high speed the whole time without ever putting the cars in for service causes wear and tear, and so if we eat constantly, we're effectively increasing the wear and tear on our bodies.

So what fasting or severely limiting energy consumed from food does is put our bodies in for a service. We deprive our body of calories (fuel) and that way, instead of making the body produce new cells, we encourage it to take stock—and take care of—the cells it already has.

IGF-1: The 1 to Watch?

IGF-1 is a growth hormone that many scientists in this field believe is central to the effects of this diet *and* to both the aging process and the development of cancers. IGF-1 stands for Insulin-Like Growth Factor and it plays an important role in children's growth. But once we're adults, the effects are not as positive: in particular, the hormone seems to lock us into this constant cycle of regrowth that may not do us any favors—the go-go mode Dr. Mosley talked about.

There's firm evidence in animal studies that lower levels of IGF-1 can lead to better health and longer life expectancy: mice on a diet of either continuous calorie restriction or intermittent calorie restriction have been shown to live 40 percent longer than mice fed a normal diet. That would be the equivalent of a person living to 120 or more!

Indeed, a recent report also suggests that in the future a hormone that blocks the action of IGF-1 might offer some of the longevity benefits of fasting or calorie restriction—without having to fast! A group of mice were genetically engineered to produce constant supplies of a hormone usually produced during fasting, FGF21. The experiment extended their life span by a third, although fertility and bone density were affected (for more detail about all these studies, refer to the links section at the back of the book).

The Curious Case of the People "Immune" to Cancer

Of course, we need to be wary of assuming that what works in mice will work in the same way for us. One clue comes from a rare human genetic condition known as Laron syndrome, where very low levels of IGF-1 are produced. It's a form of dwarfism, which restricts growth in people who have it, but the lack of the hormone also has very strong protective effects against cancer and diabetes. Professor Longo from the University of Southern California—the same guy who gave us the car analogy above—monitored ninety-nine people with the condition in Ecuador with astonishing results.

To date, they've now been followed for twenty-four years, and none of them have developed diabetes, and only one has been diagnosed with non-fatal cancer. Yet 5 percent of their neighbors—with similar diets and lifestyles—have been diagnosed with diabetes and 17 percent had cancer diagnosed during that same period. Overall, the Laron syndrome group didn't live longer, but that may be down to the high number of accidents caused by the practical difficulties of living in a world designed for taller people.

One thing that points toward the possible protective effects of low-levels of IGF-1 came when the scientists studied blood serum from those with the Laron mutation under a microscope. Cells suffered less DNA damage than "normal" blood cells from non-Laron patients when they were exposed to a toxin. Yet when the scientists added IGF-1, that protection disappeared.

Food and IGF-1

So if IGF-1 is a contributor to DNA damage—the kind we talked about when we were discussing free radicals and oxidative stress—then what happens when we eat less and consequently produce less IGF-1? It seems that as levels of the hormone drop, the body goes into the repair mode we mentioned before. This amazing process is one we can trace right back to the way our ancestors lived. Their lives involved the most extreme version of fasting and feasting— Tina put it so clearly when she wrote to update her progress since she's been doing 5:2.

> *If you think about it, it's the most natural way to eat and probably how our cavemen ancestors would have survived. They'd have hunted an animal, eaten their kill, and may not have caught another for a few days so would have eaten much fewer calories until their next catch.* —Tina, 49

Our bodies adapted to such dramatic variations in food intake very efficiently—but as I said in my introduction, it means they are focused on laying down fat stores, which doesn't work for us in times of permanent plenty. So this way of eating simulates the same lifestyle—and scientists have focused on the actions of one particular gene that is key to the repair processes.

The SIRT1 Gene: Gene Genius of Anti-Aging?

That gene is called the SIRT1 gene and produces a protein, sirtuin (silent mating type information regulation 2 homolog: don't worry, there won't be a test at the end). Calorie restriction and fasting seem to activate the gene, with life-extending and anti-aging effects.

It certainly does the trick for yeast and worms. Having extra copies of this gene extends their life spans. In human-focused research, there's been attention paid to the effect of calorie restriction in activating the gene, and all the "repair mode" benefits we've been discussing in this chapter.

The theory goes that sirtuin may play a part in regulating/improving the processes we've discussed above, including apoptosis (regulated cell death), reducing damage by free radicals, and also reducing what's known as inflammatory response. That's when the body tries to protect itself from infection. It works well when you have a cut or a minor infection, and various infection-fighting cells cause inflammation including redness and swelling as they race to the location to fight the infection. But it's not good news when your body stays in this inflamed state. In fact, it's thought that chronic inflammation might be responsible for many medical conditions, including cancers, heart disease, and arthritis.

So a reduction in inflammation triggered by SIRT1 may be responsible for many of these benefits seen in animals and humans, and it can be activated by calorie restriction, including 5:2 and ADF diets. Further research is ongoing into this and into the possibility that you can also give your SIRT1 gene a kick in the pants with red wine!

The Wine Connection

The skin and seeds of grapes contain a molecule called resveratrol, and some scientists believe this might partly explain the "French paradox," in which studies have shown some French citizens live longer than other Western Europeans, despite diets high in fat. But before you crack open the Merlot, you should know the research is ongoing. Billions of dollars are being spent trying to use this knowledge to develop life-extending treatments. Yet the role of the resveratrol—and the SIRT1 gene in general—in increasing life spans is still controversial.

Uncertainties and Motivation

The precise mechanisms of SIRT1, resveratrol, and IGF-1 in the fasting process are still unclear, but there are numerous studies showing the potential beneficial effects of ADF and calorie restriction on different medical conditions.

Research in this area is ongoing, but for me (and for most of the scientists involved), there's enough evidence from different sources to feel convinced that the 5:2 (or 4:2, 6:1, or ADF) life is the way forward.

In the next section, I'll summarize some of the most exciting medical research. I've found this very motivating to flip through if the hunger pangs strike! Remember there are links to all the research in the section at the back, so you can follow up the areas that are of most interest to you.

Medical Research on Specific Conditions

Much of the evidence at this stage comes from animal studies, because human life spans are so much longer and therefore the studies take longer too. So where humans have tried ADF or calorie-restricted diets, the effects are often measured by blood tests that show chemical markers. These indicate the likelihood of developing certain diseases, e.g., insulin sensitivity for diabetes or LDL and HDL cholesterol for heart disease.

The more this area of research grows, the more long-term information about the real-time results in human subjects should be available. For an excellent overview of some of the best research in the field, Dr. Krista Varady, who was featured in the *Horizon* program, and Dr. Marc Hellerstein put together a review of studies in 2007—there's a link in the resources section.

Cancer

In animal trials, there are signs that ADF (and intermittent calorie restriction) has inhibited the growth of certain cancer cells and improved response to anti-cancer therapy. Meanwhile the Genesis Breast Cancer Prevention Centre (genesisuk.org) in Manchester, England, has been measuring the effects of an intermittent calorie-restricted diet, similar to the 5:2 diet, in women with a high risk of developing the disease. Because excess weight is often associated with an increased risk of breast cancer, lowering weight can reduce the risk by up to 40 percent. But this form of dieting might offer extra benefits at a cellular level. In one study, the intermittent fasters lost nearly twice as much weight as the daily dieters and also showed greater improvements in insulin sensitivity—which is an excellent result in terms of diabetes prevention (see more about this later in the chapter).

The BRRIDE (Breast Risk Reduction Intermittent Diet Evaluation) study has analyzed breast and body tissues to see if the diet has made changes to how the genes are behaving. The hope is that a diet of 1,800 calories five days a week and 600 calories two days a week may reduce the activity of the SCD (stearoyl-CoA desaturase) gene, which is thought to be a factor in the development of certain cancer cells, including those in some breast tumors.

As I've mentioned before, most of my female relatives on my mother's side of the family have had breast cancer diagnoses. Apart from my regular mammograms, I've felt powerless in the face of this history. Until now. The evidence may not yet be there in black and white, but I await the outcome of this study with particularly keen interest. Dr. Michelle Harvie and her Genesis team have also written a new book summarizing their dietary advice. There are full details on this, and all the research in this chapter, in the resources section at the end of the book.

Prevention is, obviously, better than a cure, but there are also indications from research in animals and some limited studies of humans that fasting at the right time can make chemotherapy treatment easier to tolerate, and perhaps more successful. One theory is that fasting puts the body's healthy cells into the slower-paced repair mode, but the "rogue" cancer cells are still proliferating. So the healthy cells are less vulnerable to the toxic effects of chemotherapy, while the malignant cells that the chemo is targeting are attacked more effectively. Research in this area is ongoing as I write, and any decisions about fasting before such treatment must be discussed with your oncology team.

Heart Disease

Cardiovascular disease affects almost every family. It's the leading cause of death in the UK and worldwide. The term is used more broadly than you might think, and it may include high blood pressure, heart attacks, and also strokes, so it's understandable that it's a major concern. It's also one of the areas of medicine that researchers are focusing on when they're assessing the benefits of fasting diets.

In animal studies, rodents saw a decrease in blood pressure, heart rate, and cardiovascular disease risk indicators when they were put on ADF regimens. In another experiment on rats, the damage caused when a heart attack was induced was less in those on ADF.

Krista Varady and her team at the University of Illinois have led the research with human subjects in this field. She has run a number of studies (find more details in the resources section), which have shown that intermittent fasting is effective in helping people lose weight, and the diet also appears to result in less loss of muscle than conventional calorie-controlled diets. The important results for cardiovascular health were the reduction in levels of LDL (or "bad") cholesterol and triglycerides in the blood, and lower blood pressure readings were also reported in one study.

In our initial small group of 5:2 dieters, six have already reported lower blood pressure readings and several more have seen lower levels of bad cholesterol.

Type-2 Diabetes

I've seen first-hand how type-2 (or "late onset") diabetes is not the minor inconvenience many people assume it to be. The condition can cause cardiovascular problems, kidney disease, damage to the retina, nerve problems, and damage to circulation in the legs and feet that can even lead to amputation.

Type-2 diabetes is increasing dramatically in adults all across the world, but more children and young people are being diagnosed with it too, mainly due to the increase in obesity levels. The implications for the health of individuals—and the cost for health care—are frightening.

Type-2 diabetes develops when the body becomes less efficient at dealing with the sugars that we consume through food. When we eat, much of the food is turned into simple sugars that provide energy to the cells. The hormone insulin, produced by the pancreas, helps to regulate blood sugar levels. Having too much sugar in your blood is dangerous, so insulin sends an instruction to the cells to take in more glucose, so the sugar levels in the blood will drop.

The problem comes when the pancreas stops producing enough insulin or when the cells stop being as responsive or sensitive as they should be to the hormone. This happens most frequently in people who are overweight, because excess weight makes it harder for the body to regulate blood sugar, but it can also happen in those of normal weight.

For many years, dieting wisdom has favored "grazing" as a way of keeping blood sugar stable. The idea is that you snack between meals, so your blood sugar levels are never allowed to drop (a drop will send hunger signals to the brain, prompting you to eat more). This idea can work if you eat healthy food in small portions, but as we've seen, the temptations to snack on high-fat and sugary foods are great. This means you put on weight and your pancreas has to work overtime. It seems to make sense to me, as a non-scientist, that reducing the number of sugar/insulin spikes you experience by eating less often during the day would make it easier to regulate blood sugar levels.

Blood sugar levels can also affect levels of fat, because insulin is lipogenic. While insulin is circulating, your body lays down fat stores, instead of burning fat—another reason why dieters would want to reduce too many spikes. This should be exactly what intermittent fasting does: if we choose to go without food, our body will turn to getting its energy from stored sources.

So what does the research say? Animal studies (particularly on rats) certainly suggest that fasting may have a positive effect on how they process glucose, though not all human trials show the same results. However, the Genesis cancer study outlined above found that women who followed an intermittent calorie restriction regimen showed greater improvements in their insulin sensitivity than those who followed a traditional diet. Another study showed that fasting, without reducing the total number of calories consumed, made the body more responsive to insulin.

There is still more work to be done, but of course, simply losing body fat reduces the risk of type-2 diabetes. So if fasting helps you do that, it will also cut your risk or help you control diabetes if you have already been diagnosed with it.

Asthma, Auto-Immune Disorders, and Other Chronic Conditions

Numerous other studies are underway to measure the effect of intermittent fasting on conditions that affect our quality of life.

Dr. James Johnson, whose book *The Alternate-Day Diet* offers a version of intermittent fasting, has carried out research on people with asthma undertaking his diet, and he found that nineteen out of twenty people who followed it saw improvements in their symptoms. He also studied over 500 people who've followed his Alternate Day regimen. The subjects reported a range of improvements to conditions including "insulin resistance, asthma, seasonal allergies, infectious diseases of viral, bacterial and fungal origin, autoimmune disorder (rheumatoid arthritis), osteoarthritis, symptoms due to CNS inflammatory lesions (Tourette's, Meniere's), cardiac arrhythmias (PVCs, atrial fibrillation), menopause-related hot flashes."

Certainly, members of our 5:2 group have seen improvements in a number of long-standing health concerns, ranging from asthma, to hormonal problems like pre-menstrual syndrome and perimenopausal symptoms, through to joint inflammation and restless leg syndrome.

Weight is coming off, I look better in clothes and the rheumatoid arthritis in my hands doesn't hurt

*so much, and I have more movement in my fingers
without them cracking. Will be interested to see
how the blood pressure is when I see the doctor
next.   —Anita, 51*

*I had some quite severe menopausal problems and
whilst I did not particularly expect the diet to make any
difference, it was a nice surprise to find that it does. My
night sweats have stopped and whilst I get the occasional
hot flush, they're not nearly as bad as they were.
—Sally, 49*

Anecdotal evidence, of course, but I am sure there will be more to come as 5:2 and intermittent fasting grow in popularity.

For many years, medical research tended to assume that female bodies worked the same as male ones, so they carried out research on men and applied the findings to both. There's more recognition now that this can lead to false conclusions, and there are specific concerns around whether women—especially during their fertile years—may not respond in the same positive ways to ADF or intermittent calorie restriction. Sleep disturbance and a reduction in fertility have been noted in both sexes but especially in females. It's not surprising—fasting is stressful to the body (though it's good stress when it's controlled) so sleep may be harder and reproduction is not top priority if your body is primed to focus on survival. It does mean that 5:2 may not be advisable if you're trying to conceive, though of course, losing weight before trying can increase your chances of a healthy pregnancy if you are overweight.

The more aware we are of the possible pros as well as cons of this diet, the better. Of course, it has to be a personal decision but there are relevant links in the resources section.

What about Starvation Mode?

Over the years, the idea of "starvation mode" has been a scary prospect for all dieters; as I said in my diary entry, friends mentioned it to me when I began this diet. The concern is that if the body is deprived of food for a lengthy period, it will take emergency action, effectively "rationing" the number of calories it uses and becoming so efficient in using them that if you then go back to eating normally, you will put more weight on because your body is being overly efficient.

In other words, starvation mode might have protected Stone Age man (and woman!) from premature death, but it might also stop twenty-first century man and woman from ever fitting into those skinny jeans.

It's very hard to work out what's fact and what's fiction when it comes to this "mode." Some diet gurus refer to it as a myth, others hold it up as the bogeyman of dieters. A human body deprived of food for a long time—seventy-two hours or more, though opinions vary—will begin to break down cells to produce what it needs, and that's likely to mean muscle mass will decrease the longer the starvation lasts. That's not a good thing.

The key words here appear to be "lengthy period," which is the beauty of the 5:2 approach. Not only does intermittent calorie restriction help with willpower—you only have to resist temptation till you're back *off* the diet tomorrow—it also prevents any real risk of counter-productive changes to your metabolism because you're not restricting calories for long enough to (non-medical term here) freak your body out. Which has to be good news for your hard-working cells—and your health overall.

Body—and Mind

The research is impressive and exciting. But is that going to be enough to boost your willpower when you're craving chocolate at 4 in the afternoon?

Possibly. But luckily, fasting also has powerful effects on your brain, your mood, and your attitude toward food. In Chapter Four, I'll explore these in much more detail. But first, the next installment of my diet diary. I've got one fast under my belt—now what about the rest of my life?

📋 Kate's 5:2 Diary Part Three

August & September 2012

MyFitnessPal Keeps Shouting at Me
Mood: Excited, Curious, Lucky

So. One fast down, the rest of my life to go.

The day after my first Fast Day feels amazing, and I must admit I go a bit over the top on the food. The TV show says you can eat pretty much what you want on your non-diet days so . . . well, I behaved myself till teatime, even cutting the portion size of my yogurt breakfast. But then it all went a bit "thank God it's Friday night, now let's eat everything in the fridge."

I started well, with a blueberry and yogurt breakfast at just 104 calories, then had a panini at lunchtime. But at dinner it was a different story…

Italian Rose Wine, 500 ml: 300 cals

Millionaire's Shortbread Dessert: 440 cals

Tortilla Chips, 25 g: 119 cals

Edamame, Pea, and Wasabi Dip, 125 g: 208 cals

Whole Wheat Roll: 155 cals

Garlic Mushrooms, 100 g: 135 cals

Cherry Tomatoes, 5 tomatoes, 60g: 15 cals

Country Life Butter, 10 g: 69 cals

Graze Box, Toffee Apple: 68 cals

TOTAL: 1,910 CALS

I'm a bit ashamed to post it all. There's a dessert here that almost totaled my entire calorie consumption yesterday plus I had almost two-thirds of a bottle of wine (am I celebrating not being on a Fast Day?).

And yet, I need to be honest: we all have our bad days and it still came to only a little bit more than the 1876, which is what I'd worked out I could eat without gaining any more weight.

I'm definitely not going to monitor all of my Feast Days, but it's almost reassuring to know that on this diet I can eat all of those rather yummy things—now and then—and still potentially lose weight if I am careful on the Fast Days. Speaking of which,

Fast Day 2 is a Saturday . . .

. . . and I eat exactly the same as I ate on the first Fast Day. Which I thought would be boring but is actually pretty liberating. What's wrong with sticking to a breakfast option that is tasty and you know will stop you from feeling ravenous?

The schoolmarm in my computer

MyFitnessPal is quite upset with me. On Fast Day, it tells me off for eating too little, saying I might go into starvation mode. Luckily, all I've read about the science says that one day's fasting at a time won't affect my metabolism.

The strangest thing is that I've begun to like my Fast Days, even look forward to them. I feel it's a day off from thinking about food, and also a bit of a "rest" for my body, which seems to fit in with what the program said—your body repairs itself while it's not running quickly on protein.

I've been experimenting with eating at different times. With so much diabetes in my family, I'm interested in the effects of insulin and it strikes me that part of the benefit of fasting might be that your body isn't having to produce insulin all the time. So maybe trying to eat fewer meals a day is a good idea?

Hunger? Bring it on!

Just as strange is how hunger feels. I'd forgotten. Often what I'd mistaken for hunger is actually thirst or even boredom.

But now that I let myself get hungry on my Fast Days, it's not nearly as scary or overwhelming of an experience as I feared. I'm aware that I am so lucky that I can avoid food for one or two days a week without worrying whether the food will be there when I want it to be. Eating less feels like a check-in, a reminder of what the right amount is to eat and how fortunate I am that there will be food when I'm ready.

August is party month!

I knew when I decided to embark on the diet that August wasn't going to be easy. I had lots of parties and events to go to, and so I reasoned that my diet was A) going to be hard to follow and B) probably more about not packing on the pounds than helping me lose any weight. In total, I fasted on seven days this month, and my expectations were realistic.

Weight on August 31: 156 lbs

Total Lost: 5 lbs

Days on Diet: 22

Hooray! That's a bigger loss than I was expecting. My clothes are looser, and my confidence that I can lose weight this way is increasing. Could this be what I've been looking for at last?

Souped-up September

Party month over—now it's back to reality. I like autumn, and I like the chance to give the diet a proper go now. The 5 pounds I lost last month is a great start, and it also feels sustainable.

I'm now settling into a routine: Fast Days are Mondays and Wednesdays, so my weekends are free for eating out and enjoying myself without calorie counting.

I'm also skipping breakfast on my Fast Days, except for black coffee. And although I love to cook, on Fast Days I rely on very simple foods: salads, ready-made soups, perhaps some berries or yogurt. But it also means I can plan to enjoy doing some baking on the weekends, something that was completely out of bounds when I was on a low-carb diet or calorie counting all the time. But on 5:2, I'm hardly doing any calorie counting now, even on my Fast Days. I'm using MyFitnessPal sometimes, but I'm getting to know by instinct what the right level of food is.

Beet power

The weather changed midmonth, and I worried about switching from salads to relying on soup. So I experimented with the chunkier ones you buy in cans in the supermarket. Even the ones with cheese or cream rarely contain more than 150 calories per portion, so they could form the basis of my food for the day. I rather like that most of my food is contained in one can: it makes Fast Days look less daunting somehow.

One of my favorite choices is beet soup. I'm surprised I haven't turned beet pink as my Fast Days often include some of the red peril—especially the marinated spicy beet from my local store that I eat by the bucket load. Still, whatever works for me, right?

On top of my daily soup ration, there's room for a couple of 100-calorie snacks or treats: beets(!), some frozen berries with yogurt and a tiny amount of muesli for texture, a couple of apples, a banana, and the world's smallest portion of tortilla chips. One evening I had plans to meet friends and didn't want to cancel, so I even allowed myself a 100-calorie glass of wine. It did seem a bit decadent to use a fifth of my calories on alcohol, but at least I'm a cheap date.

The dollhouse portions are slightly surreal and maybe a bit sad-looking on even the smallest plates I have in the house, but because it's only a couple of days a week, I don't care too much. I can see how the measuring and weighing could become an obsession, and not an altogether healthy one, which is why I think the days when you eat what you like are important for psychological, as well as physiological, reasons. It's about enjoying the pleasure of food, which is so often absent in a diet.

Feasting not feeding!

I've decided to call my eating days "Feast Days." On the TV show, they called them "feed days," which had a slightly barnyard feel about it and also reminded me a bit of an article I'd read about "feeders"—men who like to date larger women and watch as they eat a lot. Those two ideas aren't really fitting in with my hopes for this lifestyle, whereas "feast" feels far better. The point is not to indulge in a frenzy of cakes and puddings, but to savor the food on the days when you're free to eat what you like.

I also find that the early tendency to overdo it slightly on my Feast Days is reducing as I get used to the diet. One reason is that after counting the calories the day before, I am more aware of what everything contains, so a chocolate brownie is something I choose to savor after a small lunch rather than something I scarf down unnoticed as I run for the train. And it tastes so good! The other reason is that all your senses are heightened after a day of fasting. Even a single slice of toast with peanut butter feels like a feast after a day when I've managed just fine on fewer than 500 calories.

Weight on 30 September: 152 lbs

Total Lost: 9 lbs

Days on Diet: 52

I slowed down a little so it's still not a dramatic weight loss, but at this rate, I should have lost almost 20 pounds by Christmas and be back into the healthy-BMI zone.

It might not seem like a huge breakthrough, but it really is. When I remember how I felt in July—that my weight and my attitude toward food were out of control, that I had no way of "stopping the rot"—I feel very lucky.

And, of course, I'm seeing the difference. My clothes are looser and even my bra needs adjusting. Could the dreaded back fat be facing its nemesis?
Bring it on, October!

The Hunger Game— Fasting Is Good for the Brain

Reading my diary after a few months on the diet, it strikes me even more forcefully how important the right mental attitude is to increasing the chances of succeeding at any lifestyle change, particularly weight loss.

Or at least, people who are successful at losing weight are those who have the mental strength to ignore cravings for long-term physical benefit. It's something I know many dieters—including me—find difficult. If the body showed the results of that slice of chocolate cake overnight, it might be easier.

As we've established, our bodies are built to consume and conserve energy for survival. Pretty vital for early humans, but in the industrialized twenty-first century, when many of us are lucky enough to have a vast choice and availability of food, making the "right" choices about what we consume can be easier said than done. In theory, we have lots of appetizing fresh produce available and can make the right decisions. In practice, I know many of us feel out of control.

If you read the diary entries I've included in this book, you'll get a sense that my own weight issues result from a whole cocktail of factors:

- switching from an active job to a sedentary one;
- hating most forms of exercise;
- a sweet tooth, and a savory one;
- a love of cooking, especially baking;
- a slightly addictive personality;
- a naturally, um, curvy body shape;
- a strong association between food and reward.

Which means that whenever I'm feeling a little bit bad about how tight my jeans are, my first instinct is to head straight for the cookie jar.

What's Your Reason?

How about you? Why not take a couple of minutes to think about the reasons you might not be making the right choices? Do any of these ring a bell?

Stress: We lead busy lives, commute long distances, and work long hours, so often we turn to food—particularly dishes high in fat or sugar—to provide fast energy boosts to meet a deadline or comfort ourselves after a hard day.

Commercial interests: Manufacturers and retailers know that processed foods often generate higher profits, so these are marketed in ways that promote those energy-boosting or comforting qualities. It's often easier to buy "comfort" foods or fast food when we're on the move than to try to buy or prepare fresher or unprocessed foods.

Mixed messages: It can be hard to determine which foods are healthy when some foods labeled "low-fat" turn out to be high in sugar, or vice versa.

Media images of beauty: Photographs, including those that are air-brushed, present such perfect human specimens that we lose sight of what normal or healthy is, and when we can't live up to the impossible, we comfort ourselves with food.

Upbringing: Our own attitudes toward food as a reward or punishment will be closely related to our upbringing and those around us, such as being offered cookies or alcohol to "compensate" for someone doing something unpleasant, or experiencing conflict.

Hunger phobia: We are often so busy "grazing" or eating food throughout the day that we become terrified of feeling hungry even though for most of us in industrialized nations, it will only be a temporary state. Yet that constant feeding can also remove the anticipation that goes with building up to a delicious meal.

Remember How It Feels to Be Hungry?

I had forgotten until I started this diet. I often ate because I was thirsty or bored, and had totally lost touch with the basics of appetite or enjoying the anticipation before sitting down to eat.

The first days of fasting were a revelation—because I realized I could feel hungry, acknowledge it, and then carry on with my day-to-day life. I would distract myself with sparkling water, black coffee or herbal tea, or even exercise. The pangs came in bursts and if I could ignore those, then they'd subside.

The key to being able to ignore those nagging hunger pangs? I knew it would be different the next day. I knew that if I couldn't put off eating what I liked just for a few more hours until the next day (and knowing all the benefits to my body), then really there was no hope for me at all.

Willpower deserts me when a diet is never-ending. But when it's simply a matter of anticipating and enjoying my food the next day, it's so much easier. Many others agree that soon the "restriction" of a Fast Day begins to feel more like a "liberation" from worrying about food and allows the rest of your life to feel normal.

It allows me to have my Saturday night meal out and a few glasses of wine on a Friday without feeling as though I have "broken my diet." This means my

relationship with my husband doesn't have to change,
as we always eat out on Saturdays. —*Julie, 45*

Fat Crimes and Punishments

The problem I've had with previous diets has been the feeling of deprivation—even punishment—that constant calorie counting can provoke. You might recognize this: you start with the best of intentions but soon feel as though your newly restricted food intake is the penalty for being greedy. Then, in a difficult moment, you think, *Screw it, if I'm greedy, then so be it!* and console yourself with your comfort food of choice—chocolate, cheese, bread, wine—which triggers a whole new cycle of guilt.

Or you can gain a reputation as the picky one at friends' dinner parties or celebrations, which highlights the fact that you're on a diet "again" and also highlights any failures.

The 5:2 Diet changes how you view your eating habits, and the change is likely to be permanent. In fact, many people prefer not to call 5:2 a diet at all, because of the negative associations with unworkable or abandoned weight loss regimens. I use diet here because it's brief and it can also simply mean what you eat, but you may prefer to call this a plan, an approach, a way of eating, or a lifestyle to maximize the chances of making this change a permanent one.

The psychological benefits are one thing, but there also seem to be benefits at the cellular level in terms of brain function.

Effects on the Brain: Sharper and for Longer?

The *Horizon* TV program introduced me to a rather special breed of mouse, one that had been bred to develop Alzheimer's disease. Different groups of these mice were then fed different diets: some the equivalent of junk food, others as much normal food as they wanted, and then a third group was subject to "intermittent energy restriction," a day-on/day-off regimen similar to ADF. The last group was much slower to develop Alzheimer's even though they were destined to do so, and tests showed that the mice benefited from a range of changes, including an increase in levels of BDNF, a protein that helps to protect existing neurons (brain cells) and encourage the growth of new ones. The mice on the ADF-style regimen also had better memories.

Why Would Fasting Help the Brain?

But why would this be happening? Again, common sense suggests that on reduced calories, the brain would be slowing down its activity, as the cells of the body do, rather than "wasting" energy.

Neuroscientist Mark Mattson from the American National Institute on Aging believes there's a biological reason why fasting would make the brain function better: if early man couldn't find or catch food, he'd go hungry and, ultimately, die. Therefore it makes absolute sense that his brain should work harder to either discover new sources of food or remember where he found it the last time.

So, fasting stresses the nerve cells but—as we've seen with the other medical research—this stress may be good stress, improving mental fitness, just as exercise stresses the muscles to improve physical fitness.

The research has implications not only for Alzheimer's disease and other forms of dementia, but also strokes. Professor Mattson is now planning more research on humans to see whether fasting can stave off age-related cognitive decline. There are indications that the greatest benefits start at middle age, so it may be that beginning this way of eating before that stage of life has less significant results.

The practical difficulties of research into the brain— not the least of which is that changes can often only be detected in patients when an autopsy is carried out after death—mean conclusive evidence on some of these areas will take time. But Mattson himself reportedly switched from a calorie-restricted diet to intermittent fasting, and many more experts in this field are adopting the lifestyle with the same enthusiasm *they* show in their research.

Mood and Energy Boosts— the Biggest Surprise of All

I hate it when the clocks go back. I don't suffer from Seasonal Affective Disorder, the depressive symptoms many people experience during the winter months, but my mood and energy levels are definitely affected by the dark and cold. I can be a bit of an Eeyore, to put it mildly.

It was one of the coldest, bitterest winters in the UK this year, yet I felt more energetic than I did in the summer, and was almost irritatingly positive. When I looked back at my diary entries, I noticed that had been an upward trend since I started the diet.

I'd assumed this was because I was feeling good about my weight loss, but even so it seemed particularly notice-able. And then I read Dr. Mosley's new book, *The Fast Diet*, which offers advice based on his excellent program and also expands on some of the science. In it, he mentions that Mark Mattson believes these better moods may be due to increased levels of the BDNF protein caused by fasting.

I was fascinated, so I followed up. I've found plenty more evidence, including studies that show stress can decrease BDNF levels in the brains of rats with adverse effects on parts of the brain that are also affected in humans suffering from chronic depression. Anti-depressant medications and even electroconvulsive therapy have been shown to reverse this decrease. So if fasting is doing the same, this could be incredibly exciting for those with a history of depressive ill-ness. It may also be one of the reasons the experience of fasting can be so uplifting even for those who don't suffer. Interestingly, exercise can also reverse age-related declines in BDNF levels, and many of us who fast have seen our energy and inclination to exercise increase too.

The more I read, the more the links between so many varied diseases become clear, and the more excited I become by the work scientists like Mattson, Varady, and Longo are doing.

In Summary

5:2 and other intermittent-fasting or restriction diets can:

- Save you money
- Help you lose weight with minimal hassle
- Make it easier to maintain a healthy weight

And they may:

- Reduce your chances of developing life-threatening diseases
- Change your attitude toward food and hunger
- Help you stay mentally sharper for longer
- Boost your mood and energy levels, often dramatically

In the next part, I'll explain how to adapt this diet so it works best for you. But first, will the winter sun be my diet's undoing?

Kate's 5:2 Diary Part Four

October & November 2012

Hiccups in the Sun
Mood: Evangelical, Positive, Flexible

October

Everyone I talk to seems to know someone who is doing this diet, and it's as appealing to men as to women. I've been chatting to men about why, especially as so many men I know are reluctant to admit to dieting. Is it the all-or-nothing nature of the Fast Days? The simplicity of it? Or maybe it's just that it *really* works?

I've also set up a page on Facebook called *The 5:2 Diet* so we can share our experiences. But the Facebook group is only the start. I feel so evangelical about this plan that I've decided to write all I know about it as a book, the book I wish there'd been when I first heard about the diet.

OK, I'm not a scientist, but I did work as a journalist on news, documentaries, and food programs at the BBC for fifteen years, so I'm pretty used to separating fact from fiction. Plus, I've learned a huge amount about how the diet works in real life by talking to others who are doing it.

The hiccups

Of course, the moment I decided to write about the diet, my weight loss stalled. I lost nothing in the first week of writing and felt slightly disheartened. There's a second hiccup on the horizon: I'm off on vacation to Tenerife for a week this month, and I know I won't be fasting there, so I decided on a pre-emptive strike, switching to ADF—fasting every other day— for the week beforehand.

Again, I was surprised how easy it was. I simply fell into a routine of eating well but unrestrictedly one day and then being extra careful the next. I hardly weigh any foods out anymore but am grateful for "gourmet" fresh soups. I know how cheap it is to make your own, but it also involves being tempted to add little extras to the recipe, whereas these cans involve no more preparation than pressing a button on the microwave.

Cheap as fries

Despite buying ready-made soups, I'm saving money through this diet. In fact, I must remember to stop buying as many groceries as my freezer won't fit all the things I've been buying but then don't eat.

I'm cutting back on my snacking on Fast Days but also on Feast Days because I am somehow more able to ask myself the question, "Do I really want this?" If I do, then it's absolutely fine. But even being able to ask that question seems to curb my appetite.

And on the Fast Days I am eating very little, so my shopping bill has gone down, unlike when I was low-carb dieting and had to buy lots of expensive protein, or when I was doing normal calorie counting and spent a fair amount on special "low-cal" options that always cost more.

There are occasional moments of comedy too, like the day I took a french fry off my boyfriend's plate, then insisted on weighing a similar-sized one and entering it into MyFitnessPal. One fry = 8 calories = too much!

A week off-track

I don't count a single calorie on vacation. Buffet breakfasts, buffet dinners, and lots of lovely Spanish wine. Buffets are notoriously bad news for dieters. I've read about research that shows the variety makes us go a bit crazy, grabbing a little bit of this and that and the other, which adds up to far more calories than we'd eat at a normal meal. But I am more conscious of stopping when I am hungry, not least because my bikini body is still not as svelte as I'd like it to be.

With that in mind I do something unprecedented: go the hotel gym! Four times. It's not easy because the weather is hot and the gym's not air-conditioned and the equipment is pretty basic, but I do it. Everyone else in the gym is very buff and I feel a bit like the lardy girl in the corner. But maybe before long I'll be buff too?

> Weight on October 31st: 150lbs
> Total Lost: 11lbs
> Days on Diet: 83
> BMI: 25.9 (which means I'm within a point of a healthy BMI)
> OK, it's only a loss of 2 pounds this month but I have had a great vacation, plus I think I am putting on muscle from the gym.
>
> As for my goal, well, till now I haven't dared have one, but I think I'd like to be a nice round (well, not that round) 10 stone [140 pounds], or maybe 9 stone 13 [139 pounds] to be in single figures.

November: Back to fasting and feasting

I loved my vacation, but I did look forward to coming back to my food routine. I like the thought that it's doing me good as well as making me look better in my clothes. So after I get back, I switch from 5:2 to 4:3. I started again with ADF—roughly, it's probably more like three Fast Days a week—and deliberately didn't weigh myself in the week or so after I returned from vacation because I didn't want to feel downhearted. But my jeans are still looser than they were.

My routine is pretty fixed now, but I'm experimenting with exercise. I did join the gym just before I started this lifestyle, but it's become more important to me while I'm doing this. At first, I avoided exercising on a Fast Day, but recently I've tried it and it's fine for me. I don't feel noticeably dizzy or wobbly if I do it. And the exercise just feels like part of what I want to do to look after myself more and maximize the benefits of the diet. I also don't eat any more to compensate for the calories I've burned at the gym. Once I do an extra-long workout—burning around 500 calories—and eat 470, that puts me into a strange minus calories place on MyFitnessPal. . . . And makes me feel very smug.

The eggs Florentine episode

The one thing with this way of eating is that it can be slightly less than sociable. It's easy to schedule the diet for a couple of days a week when you have nothing planned, but 4:3 or ADF means you have to fast on Friday, Saturday, or Sunday, which are the days we often do something spontaneous.

That's what happened on Sunday. We went to my favorite café, and I thought, *That's fine, I'll have the soup.*

Then came the bombshell—they don't serve soup on weekends!

There was nothing on the menu that seemed likely to be under 500 calories. Their breakfasts are legendary, their cakes towering, and I was seriously grumpy as I ordered black coffee and braced myself to watch everyone else scarfing breakfast.

"This is very antisocial," said my boyfriend. "And perhaps a little obsessive. After all, it's only one day. One meal."

I tried to think about the counterarguments—the fact that the Fast Days do involve commitment. And yet he did have a point . . .

So I went and ordered the eggs Florentine—two poached eggs, spinach, sourdough toast, and (this is the only unhealthy bit) lashings of sunshine-yellow hollandaise sauce—vowing that I'd scrape off the sauce, even though it's my favorite part.

And then I inhaled the whole thing.

At home, I looked up hollandaise on MyFitnessPal. When I've tried to make it myself, it involved vast quantities of butter. So yes, it was high fat and very calorific. But so what if I'd gone over on one of my Fast Days? It's one day in my life. What this diet is doing is making me aware and informed about what I put in my body.

The Eggs Florentine Episode is a warning not to take it too seriously. To live a little.

And, guess what? I didn't actually feel hungry for the rest of the day.

Every day I write the book

I've spent the month working on the 5:2 book. Researching the science and talking to dozens of other people doing this has made me even more enthusiastic about what we're all doing. My only frustration is that I didn't discover this years ago.

Weight on November 30: 145 pounds
Total Lost: 16 pounds
BMI: 24.9 (In the healthy range, hooray!)
Days on Diet: 113

Well, I knew something good was happening since I've already swapped from my old baggy size 14 jeans back for the 12s, and even they feel loose. But it's lovely to see that reflected on the scale. Plus, my energy levels are so high that I'm actually feeling festive, something very rare for me as the nights get longer!

Christmas? Bring it on!

PART TWO
5:2 YOUR WAY

Planning and Personalizing for Success

Step One: How Much Do You Want to Lose, and How Much Can You Afford to Eat?

The Freedom to Make Fasting Work for You

So you know the theory and science behind the diet—now it's time to work out what you want to achieve with this approach to eating, and to make some plans.

Unlike all the other diets I've tried over the years, 5:2 is completely flexible—you can even choose not to do 5:2 at all, but to try 4:3, 6:1, or whatever combination fits your life. It's one of the reasons it's so sustainable.

This section outlines three steps:

1. **Planning** what you want from this way of eating, and how you'll achieve it.

2. Fasting for the first time—with lots of tips and ideas to make it as easy as possible.

3. Reviewing what works for you, including tips on exercise, weigh-ins, and Feast Days!

Prepare for some math. I'll keep them to a minimum, but the calculations will help you plan and monitor your progress.

Even if you're attracted to 5:2 for health reasons, rather than weight loss, it's worth doing some measuring now, to help you see what changes it's making.

There's so much more to this than numbers—it's about how you feel and look, and how well your body's working—but if you want to fine-tune the diet, don't skip this part. The good news is that it should take you no time at all to work the figures out, and once you have, you're all set.

Goal Setting: Where Do You Want to Be?

Weigh Yourself. Yes, I know. If you're worried about your weight, this part is grim. But once you begin to lose weight, you'll be glad you've been honest with yourself at this stage, because your progress will be all the more impressive.

Calculate Your BMI

As you read in "The Math of Weight Loss" chapter, BMI isn't always the best indicator of what your weight means for you—especially if you're very athletic—but it does give a basic indicator. Here's a refresher on the math; you calculate it using this simple formula:

$$\text{BMI} = [(\text{Weight in pounds}) / (\text{Height in inches} \times \text{Height in inches})] \times 703$$

Or even more simply by using the calculator on any number of weight loss websites; just search for "BMI calculator."

The alternative measurement I outlined in "The Math of Weight Loss" chapter is your height/waist ratio, which is increasingly seen by doctors as more useful than BMI in predicting the chance of cardiovascular problems (for an explanation, refer back to that chapter).

First, measure your waist. Ideally, you want the measurement to be less than half of your height. You can monitor your progress by dividing your waist size by your height—if your waist gets smaller, than so will the ratio.

As an example, here's how mine has changed before and after 5:2.

August 2012: Waist (32 inches) ÷ Height (64 inches) = 0.5
January 2013: Waist (29.5 inches) ÷ Height (64 inches) = 0.46

My only comment on using this as your only progress check is that it's likely to be slower to change than weight loss, so it may not be as immediately motivating. Plus, as I've always had quite a pear shape, my starting measurement was (just) acceptable yet I was clearly overweight. So although that measurement indicated a low-ish risk of cardiovascular problems, I knew my weight was putting me at higher risk of diabetes, given how common it is in my family.

So I suggest keeping a record of BMI, weight, *and* waist measurement, and then choosing a single goal to focus on. You could express that as a BMI, a goal in pounds, or a waist measurement ratio.

For example for me, my goal weight was 9 stone 13 [139 pounds], which is A) in single figures when it comes to stones, just (!) and B) represented a BMI of 23.83.

Your goal may not be this clear if you're not aiming to lose weight, but it's still worth doing these, particularly if you're already lean. You don't want to slip into the under-weight category as that too can have negative health implications. If you monitor yourself, you can make adjustments to how often you fast, e.g. moving from 5:2 to 6:1 with just one fasting day a week or increasing your calorie consumption on Feast Days.

Diet Calculations: How to Reach Your Goal

How many days a week can you fast/calorie restrict?

The diet is called 5:2 by many because the ratio of 5 "normal" days and 2 "diet" days works really well for most people—it offers weight loss, but it's manageable in terms of finding quieter days when it works to eat less and also means you don't feel like you're on a diet most of the time.

But other options for weight loss include 4:3 (with 3 Fast Days) or Alternate Day Fasting (ADF). Here's a selection of how the choices our dieters have made suit them.

Every other day—500 calories. —Sally, 49

I follow standard 5:2, but probably consume 700 to 800 calories on Fast Days (but I'm tall and exercise a lot). —James, 43

Two days, and I aim for about 600 calories a day as I don't need to lose weight. —Nina, 52

Two days. 300 calories. —Sarah, 37

Of course, the more often you fast, the faster you'll lose. For those mainly seeking the health benefits without weight loss, 6:1 seems to be the preferred option.

How Much Should You Eat on This Diet?

Fast Days (the "2" in the 5:2 Diet) are when you're restricting your calorie intake to approximately 25 percent of your daily calorie requirement (DCR).

I've outlined how to calculate your DCR below, because I wanted to do that myself. But since the first edition of this book, I've realized most people prefer to stick to the averages, which is much easier and works very effectively for most people.

The average active woman needs approximately 2,000 calories per day. So your goal intake for Fast Days is 500.

Active men need on average 2400 calories a day so they get an extra 100 calories, or a goal intake of 600 calories.

Still want to find your own precise goal? It's easy as ABC and may give you a higher goal, particularly if your BMI is very high and you have a lot of weight to lose.

Stage A: What a Girl (or Guy) Needs

You begin by working out your Basal Metabolic Rate—how many calories someone of your size, height, and age needs just to get through the day. That is, to keep your most basic functions going. There are two different formulas: the Harris Benedict and the Mifflin St. Jeor: the latter takes age into account so that's the one I've included.

Mifflin St. Joer:

Male: BMR = (4.5 x weight in pounds)
+ (15.87 x height in inches)
- (5 x age) + 5

Female: BMR = (4.5 x weight in pounds)
+ (15.87 x height in inches)
- (5 x age)–161

It's *much* easier to use an online calculator, but if you prefer to do the math by hand, you can use the formulas above. As an example, a fifty-year-old man who is 5 feet 10 inches tall and weighs 196 pounds has an estimated BMR of 1,755 calories per day.

Stage B: Factor in Your Activity Level

The BMR sounds low—so now we factor in how active you are, to give a truer estimate of your actual Daily Calorie Requirements. This factor is the same for men and women.

Little/no exercise: BMR x 1.2 = Total Calorie Need

Light exercise: BMR x 1.375 = Total Calorie Need

Moderate exercise (3–5 days/week): BMR x 1.55 = Total Calorie Need

Very active (6–7 days/week): BMR x 1.725 = Total Calorie Need

Extra active (exercise and physical job): BMR x 1.9 = Total Calorie Need

You can use online calculators for this too, but it's a simple calculation. Our male dieter in the example above does limited light exercise, so we multiply his BMR by 1.375, so:

$$1755 \times 1.375 = \text{DCR of 2,413 calories}$$

Stage C: Lower, Lower!

So to maintain his weight, our male dieter could eat up to 2,413 calories. But he's fasting to lose weight and for the health benefits, so on Fast Days he needs to eat a quarter of his DCR.

$$2413 \div 4 = 603 \text{ calories}$$

Is It Worth It?

So, after all that math, we've ended up very close to the 600 average goal for men. It's up to you whether you want to go with the prescribed averages or do the calculations yourself. As I've said, if you're heavier, you may find this gives you a few extra calories to play with. In my case, as I record in my diary, I "lost" 30 calories as my goal was 469, but I suspect my weight loss would have been pretty much the same had I aimed at 500.

If you make these calculations and then lose a lot of weight, you'll want to recalculate, because your calorie requirement decreases as your weight does—UNLESS you step up your levels of activity, which may well happen as you find you have more energy and confidence.

So that's the math. Time to tailor the diet to suit you!

Which Day(s) Do I Fast?

Picking the right days will improve your chances of success. The first time(s) you fast, you're likely to feel hungry at first, with possible other side effects like headaches, or feeling cold or slightly light-headed. Most become used to this very quickly, but it makes sense to schedule your first couple of Fast Days for days when you have fewer commitments and can afford to take it a little easier. Though it's best not to clear your calendar completely—most people have found that staying busy is the best distraction from any hunger pangs.

Choose days when you have no social engagements or don't have to be around people who might be skeptical or try to persuade you to give up. If you are responsible for family meals, try to build in days when the meal is healthier and you can have a small portion without attracting too much attention. I like to do my Fast Days when my partner is working late or socializing with friends because that way I won't be tempted to eat what he's eating at home!

It can be useful to have regular days, e.g. Monday and Wednesday, because you can schedule around them. At first, I didn't exercise on Fast Days so scheduled around that. But it's your diet—feel free to experiment. I definitely find it helps to mark the Fast Days on my e-calendar and to-do lists. This way I feel that I have committed to them!

If a "whole day" fast doesn't work for you, some people fast for part-days that still add up to twenty-four hours. So you might eat a normal lunch on Monday, then stick to 500 or 600 calories until a later lunch or early supper on Tuesday evening.

When Will I Eat on My Fast Days?

You can choose to eat your calorie allowance in one, two, or even three meals, although evidence suggests that the health benefits may be higher if you restrict to one or two meals, with as little snacking as possible.

This is how Krista Varady's study worked: participants had a single, larger meal at lunchtime on their "Fast" Days. This makes sense to me because it appears to give the body less to "do" in terms of digesting food, producing insulin, etc. Dr. Mosley, by contrast, decided that he would eat two meals and it still worked for him, both in terms of weight loss and reduction in IGF-1.

At the start, I could never have imagined a whole day without any food. But five months in, I frequently eat only in the early evening on a Fast Day, to try to maximize the health benefits, and I don't find it difficult at all. Equally, if it's cold and I want some soup at lunchtime to warm myself up, I don't worry too much. And neither should you if you want to have three meals. You're still doing something great for your body.

That's the beauty of this diet compared to all the others I've tried (and abandoned): you decide how to make the diet fit your life, rather than the diet dictating how to live it. Here's how some other dieters divide up their Fast Day calorie allowances.

No breakfast. Porridge midday. Veg soup in evening.
Couple of barley cups during day and perhaps a rice
cake.   —Stephen, 47

One meal in the evening with my family. Portions
small except for green salad/veg. An entire bag of salad
is about 40 calories (a single egg is about 80 calories
and as for cheese or, god forbid, mayonnaise . . . !)
—Myfanwy, 49

I can't do just one meal a day as I need the psychological
feeling of having three meals a day.   —Nina, 52

Minding the Gap

There's another way to try to maximize the health benefits, and that's by being aware of the gap between the last meal on Feast Day and the first on Fast Day. And then doing the same when it's a Feast Day again. I do this, because it seems to make sense to increase fasting time. For example:

MONDAY FEAST DAY:
Eat dinner at 6 p.m.

TUESDAY FAST DAY:
Eat main meal at 6 p.m. (no breakfast or lunch)

WEDNESDAY FEAST DAY:
Skip breakfast, eat lunch late, e.g., 2 p.m.

Some 5:2 dieters do go for a "full" fast, where you only drink water or herbal teas. If the "gap" planning above is taken into account, you could fast completely for forty-four hours, but there would only be one day where you don't eat.

MONDAY FEAST DAY:
Eat dinner at 6 p.m.

TUESDAY FAST DAY:
Fast completely

WEDNESDAY FEAST DAY:
Skip breakfast, eat lunch late, e.g., 2 p.m.

Bear in mind that total fasts can be harder to stick to, but there are many alternatives, such as compressing your mealtimes into a small "window," so you avoid food for twenty hours and limit eating to between, say, 1 p.m. and 5 p.m. Again, this may maximize the benefits.

> *I try to postpone eating all day so I can eat in the evenings, but I'm not sure this helps much. It probably does regarding the metabolic changes needed for fat mobilization and brain growth, because the longer we go, the better it is, but it might undermine the repair-at-night side of things. The research suggested eating at midday, but I fear once I start eating I would want more.* —Linda, 52

The truth is that there isn't a study I've found comparing different fasting configurations. I am sure that will come, but in the meantime, experiment to find your best approach.

Consecutive or Nonconsecutive?

Most people schedule the days nonconsecutively as the hunger pangs can be stronger and a two-day fast can become an ordeal rather than a "mini-break." This risks making it less sustainable than the nonconsecutive option. Some doctors would also be wary of someone undertaking a fast for more than twenty-four hours without being checked thoroughly beforehand and maybe even supervised throughout.

What Will I Eat on My Fast Day?

Exactly what you like . . . so long as it doesn't exceed your calorie limit. I know 500 or 600 calories isn't a lot to play with, but take it from me, you can still make satisfying choices.

Banana for breakfast. Apple and yogurt for lunch. Chicken and salad for dinner. —Karl, 49

Loads of cups of tea with a little milk, nothing till supper, then a normal family supper with few/no carbs. —Julia, 50

All homemade food, so it's hard to work out the calories. I'll avoid carbs and alcohol and have a small helping of chicken or fish and lots of vegetables; a bowl of homemade soup and fruit for the other meal. I'm aiming to only eat between 12 and 6 p.m. too, on most other days. —Linda, 52

I stick to fruit and veg, beans on toast, soups, and Weight Watcher ready meals. —Jane, 49

There are plenty more sample menus and food ideas in the third section of the book. I do recommend planning in advance—the very last thing you want to be doing on your first Fast Day is going into the supermarket.

Obviously, it also depends on how many meals you're planning to have—it's very easy to find ready meals with 400 to 500 calories if you're only having a single meal, but it gets slightly harder if you want two or even three. That's where soups come into play—they tend to fill you up for longer with fewer calories.

I am also more careful to remember to take a multi-vitamin during the fasts, not because I think a day or two of eating less will do serious damage, but it's a good insurance policy.

How Will I Monitor What I Eat on Fast Days?

Studies suggest that dieters who keep a record of what they eat tend to be more successful, and it will help you pinpoint where you might be going wrong if you need to amend your habits or consumption. You can either do that electronically, or jot it down in a notebook.

The brilliant thing about 5:2 is that most of us only need to record what we eat on Fast Days, which is so much less hassle than daily dieting. If you're eating ready-made meals, recording your consumption can be very easy. They all have the nutritional information on the package, or you just scan the barcode if you have MyFitnessPal on your phone. Online sites allow you to keep your diary completely private, but you may find it helps to keep you motivated if you share it with others.

If you're cooking from scratch, weigh the ingredients carefully and then either use a calorie counter book or an online calorie guide to add up what you're eating. I prefer the latter because it does the math for you, and thousands of other users are constantly updating the site with new foods and brands. On top of this, you can use it to calorie-count your own recipes. It's how I've done the dishes in Part Three, for example. A digital scale is most accurate, or you can use measuring cups or spoons (so long as you don't overload them!).

At first, you'll probably be astonished at how many calories some foods contain, but you'll become used to the portion sizes you're allowed on Fast Days and it'll soon be second nature.

That's enough theory! Are you ready to try your first fast?

Step Two:
Your First Fast

Time for lift off—and weight off! The last section has prepared you so you know what and when to eat. This section is mainly about strategies and tips from those of us who have been there.

Motivation

The first Fast Day can be a roller coaster, though most of us found it way easier than we expected. The biggest motivation for many of us has been the mantra:

It's only a day—tomorrow I can eat what I feel like!

A Checklist of Practical Tips

On a practical level, there are many simple things you can try that will help you stay on track.

- If you can, avoid situations where you have to watch other people eat—or have to cook for the family. If you can't get out of doing the cooking, choose Fast Days to cook the things you really don't like and they do.

- Sugar-free chewing gum is another standby!

- Evenings can be a dangerous time for snackers. A hobby that uses your hands like knitting, sewing, or even jigsaw puzzles can keep you from raiding the cookie jar when you're watching TV.

- Don't forget to drink water! As well as eating up to your goal calorie limit, you can (and should) drink plenty of water. There's evidence that good hydration helps with fat loss.

- I like to drink sparkling water on Fast Days— somehow it's more enjoyable.

- You may also drink black coffee or tea, herbal teas, and diet drinks, although artificially sweetened drinks may still affect your blood sugar or insulin levels, which is not ideal on a Fast Day. There is also some debate about the effect that caffeine has on insulin, with some studies showing an increase in insulin sensitivity (which would be broadly good news) and others showing insulin spikes (less good news). As an espresso addict, I am sticking with my daily fixes for now, but as with all the decisions here, it's about personal choice.

- You may feel like going to bed early on the first few Fast Days. Use it as an excuse to relax!

And **REMEMBER**: *Tomorrow you can eat what you like!*

Friends and Frenemies

One question that does crop up is, *Whom should I tell?*

The advantages of telling people may be increased support from family members or friends, especially if they're following the diet themselves. It may also help you stay committed if people are asking you how it's going. However, reactions aren't always positive.

I find it embarrassing being on a fasting diet (because I know people will exclaim, "you're too thin to be doing it!"), so I don't talk about it outside our family. If I'm ever with other people on fasting days I tend to try and eat as little as possible without people noticing.
—Sarah, 37

I told a few people I was starting the fast and it both helped and hindered me. It helped because when I was a little cranky on those first couple of fasts they just took it as the diet, but it hindered because any conversation I had where we didn't agree (not an argument, just work related or otherwise) they said I wasn't being rational because I "needed to eat something," which wasn't the case as both times I had just eaten and they were not Fast Days! Be prepared for doubters as most people are brainwashed about skipping meals and "breakfast is the most important meal of the day" and

*"your metabolism will slow down" so I don't talk about
the diet anymore, I just get on with it. —Zoe, 38*

Men in particular can find it embarrassing to be on an
obvious diet. A recent survey suggested that one in three
male dieters wouldn't admit it, even to their closest friends
or family.

You may also worry about the impression a fasting diet
might give to younger people in your family, especially now
that there's so much awareness around eating disorders.

*I have three daughters and I am concerned about
setting a good example, and not making them too
faddy. So when they're around I stick to something
simple, like beans on toast, which doesn't look like a
"fasting" meal. —Mary, 50*

Group Therapy

An alternative to relying on friends or family is to form your
own support group or join one online. Our group of software company employees has definitely seen the benefits of
sharing:

*If a group of you is doing it, it really helps—especially
if you all do it on the same day. —Andrew, 42*

Lots of couples are deciding to embark on the plan
together—or often, one will notice how well their partner

is doing and join in (that actually happened to me!). A little healthy competition can make the process more interesting.

> *It helps a lot that my husband is also following it*
> *primarily for health reasons as he doesn't need to lose*
> *any more weight and is now having to try to eat a*
> *bit more on "normal" days to keep his weight from*
> *dropping further! Lucky him . . .   —Elaine, 52*

Even if you can't or don't want to get colleagues or family members involved, the Internet makes it really easy to connect with diet soul mates. Joining in with a forum can really help, because we can talk online to people who have been there and ask questions without feeling embarrassed. Our Facebook group grew from a handful to over 700 contributors and as a result we moved to a separate forum, at www.the5-2dietbook.com, and there are plenty more listed in the resources section of this book.

The Possible Side Effects

You may not experience any of these, but here are some of the more common things dieters have noticed in the early days. Jeanny is typical:

> *I have been feeling light headed and dizzy, but*
> *I'm not sure whether it is the diet as I haven't*
> *been doing it very long yet. Also, have had several*
> *headaches.   —Jeanny, 53*

Anyone who has made a change to their eating habits will know that the body can take a while to adapt—and 5:2 is no exception. Most of us have been surprised at how quickly we adapt to what seems like a huge change, but even so, you may experience some symptoms at first. Most are minor, but remember that if there's anything that seems extreme or worries you, you should contact your doctor. The main effects seem to be headaches, sleep disruption, and feeling the cold more in winter.

Headaches

These seem to be the number one symptom for people starting any new diet, and they can be caused by a variety of factors, including dehydration (much of our water consumption comes from food, so if we eat less of it, we may get thirsty), changes to blood sugar levels, or caffeine withdrawal. The blood sugar should stabilize, and I advise drinking lots of liquids to avoid dehydration. In terms of caffeine, there's no need to cut out coffee or tea, and in fact, I'd advise against doing this at a time when you're already trying something new. Just remember to count calories if you add milk or sweeteners or train yourself to like your coffee black.

Most people find headaches are reduced or eliminated after the first fast or two. If they continue, you can try varying meal times to cope with any blood sugar issues.

Sleep Disturbance

Some people do find it hard to sleep when they haven't eaten as much, and the mild stress that fasting causes can make you feel a little more hyper than usual. I chose to see this as a welcome energy boost while it lasted, but the usual advice about sleeplessness—take a long bath before bed, read rather than watch TV, try a milky drink—might be useful. A new suggestion involves eating one or two kiwi fruits an hour before going to bed; they've been proven to improve sleep quality by up to 40 percent.

Feeling Cold

I began the diet in August and didn't notice this, but winter starters have found that they can feel cold on Fast Days. Hot drinks and eating soup will help warm you up. You can also add spices to foods, e.g., chili flakes goes well with soups or baked beans. Also, ginger flavors in tea can give you a nice glow. It *will* get easier.

Other Effects Reported by Group Members

- **Irritability**: Feeling hungry may make you grumpy to begin with, though hunger pangs tend to disappear rather than get worse if you ignore the sensation. Low blood sugar might also make you snappy at first though again, this should stabilize. Try one of the lower-calorie treats in the food section— it's better to do without them in the long-term, but when you're starting out, be kind to yourself!

- **Digestive changes:** Constipation and reflux have been reported. It's worth including fiber (e.g. baked beans) or "digestive transit" yogurts like Activia in your Fast Days. One of our dieters was advised by her nurse to ask the pharmacist about gentle laxatives, though obviously these are not recommended for anything other than occasional use.

- **Cramps:** I used to get these all the time in the first few days on low-carb diets and haven't on this one. But I know some people have, and I've read about good responses to potassium, magnesium, and calcium supplements.

The Positives About Fast Days

Here's a list of things to remember if you're wavering.

- You're doing something good for your health and your body.

- You can work past hunger. It comes in waves, so make it a challenge to see how long it takes to feel better.

- It's incredibly beneficial to learn the difference between hunger, thirst, and boredom, all of which can become confused over time.

- You are making this choice, which tends to make you so much more appreciative of the fact that when the fast is over you can eat what you like . . .

- Not to mention the fact that any food you do have scheduled will be savored all the more!
- It can be a break for your mind *and* body as you focus on things other than food, though that may not kick in till you've done a few fasts.

Finally, here are some tips from our "expert" dieters.

Have a plan and measure out what 500 calories looks like. This will stop you from obsessing about food ALL day long. Thinking of what you will reward yourself with is also good. I plan to have a nice Thai meal with all those "naughty" carbs.   —Zoe, 38

Try to have breakfast as late as possible. When you eat in the morning it makes you feel like you want to eat more. I prefer to have my meals as late as I can. For snacking, try cherry tomatoes or carrots. Not many calories but filling. I prefer getting the fast days over and done early in the week—Mondays and Wednesdays. Fasting on days when you are not at work is harder as you have more temptations around.   —Sunil, 34

Find something to keep you busy well away from food (I fast on work days, if I can; hardly have time to eat there anyway), and treat yourself on non-fasting days so you don't feel deprived.   —Myfanwy, 49

Drink lots of boiled water or herbal teas on your fasting day. You'll find the flavor makes you feel as if you've eaten something. Also, if you like milk in your tea or coffee first thing in the morning and last thing at night, have it, even on fasting day. It will make you feel less as if you're being punished for something. It also helps to choose one treat that you intend to have the next day when you can eat what you want again, whether it's a bit of cake, some chocolate, a glass of wine, or a full English breakfast.   —Sally, 49

Finally, I love this cautionary tale from Myfanwy:

DON'T go food shopping on a Fast Day—last time I did I came home with a turkey (on special offer). Admittedly it was a runt of a turkey, but I don't even like turkey and I've never cooked one before in my life. The family thought it was hilarious.   —Myfanwy, 49

Ready, Steady, Fast!

And that's all there is to it.

By the end of today, you'll have finished your first fast, the first, I hope, of many that help you keep your eating in check and improve your health.

Step Three: Review, Revise, Revitalize

You did it! And once your Fast Day is done, you can enjoy the foods you love—perhaps some of the things you were craving yesterday. What are you looking forward to most?

The Day After

We've talked a lot about Fast Days, but what about Feast Days? These are times to relax and enjoy food and all the great things around it—being with friends and family, savoring the tastes, smells, and pleasures of cooking or eating out. In fact, it's not just about the food.

> *I find that I sleep much deeper on starving nights and wake up feeling more fresh than normal. Also, the sun seems brighter, the sky bluer and the song of birds more beautiful on the day after starving.   —Sunil, 34*

On Feast Days you can eat "normally"—in fact, many dieters prefer to call these "Normal Days" or "Nourishing Days"—but what does that actually mean? One of the things I've discovered since starting this lifestyle is that I did eat much more than I realized. So while my own "dollhouse portions" on Fast Days seem ludicrously small, the portions served in restaurants now often seem obscenely super-sized.

For me, the view of what a "portion" of food is has become skewed and that's one of the reasons many of us have suffered weight problems. So, although you can eat all the things you love on your normal days, there's clearly a sensible balance. This diet will re-educate you by stealth. You'll become fuller sooner, and you'll enjoy your favorite foods but perhaps not in the same quantities. It won't happen overnight but most of us who're doing this long-term have noticed the effect. It's almost like a reset button on an electronic appliance that's gone haywire—fasting has made me work properly again, still enjoying food, but eating what I need and no more.

If you are aiming to lose weight, you'll still need that calorie deficit we discussed in "The Math of Weight Loss" chapter: but the reset effect means most people don't need to calorie count on Feast Days to achieve that.

The work done by Krista Varady at the University of Illinois compared Alternate Day Fasters who ate a low-fat diet on their Feast Day, with those who ate a "normal" high-fat diet when they weren't fasting. Surprisingly—and happily—the reduction in weight and cholesterol was as good, if not better, in those participants who were encouraged to eat all their favorite dishes, including pizza and burgers. "Rebound" eating or over-compensation simply didn't happen on the Feast Days.

It's a finding backed up by the software engineers who've joined together to track their experiences on 5:2.

We have seen no difference in effect if you eat high-fat or low-fat food on non-fasting days. In fact, when some of us have been away on holiday, we have temporarily stopped and then restarted with little overall effect. —Andrew, 42

Of course, what you eat is one thing. How much is another matter. I admit that in the first week or two, I was tempted to overeat the things I loved. But that soon wore off, as it has for other 5:2 dieters. Even eating your Daily Calorie Requirement (DCR)—just under 2,000 calories in my case—feels like such a feast compared to the fasting that you probably won't feel the need to exceed it and, on many occasions, you'll eat less than you used to.

Mindful Eating

One tip while you're adapting would be to use the same tactic many of us use on the Fast Days—to eat very slowly, with no other distractions. No TV, no work, no multitasking. Savoring your food rather than shoveling it down means you'll probably be less tempted to overeat. But you certainly don't need to record what you're eating on the Feast Days.

Mindfulness, a form of meditation, can be a very useful tool in both controlling appetite and feeling positive and calm about the changes you're making. A friend recommended the website www.getsomeheadspace.com, which offers a free introductory trial of meditations as well as some really useful downloads, including one on mindful eating. There are also links in *the* resources section to interesting articles in the *Independent* and the *New York Times* about this.

What if I'm Not Losing Enough Weight?

If you have lost weight but it's slowed down, you could consider increasing from 5:2 to 4:3 or ADF to speed things along.

But if you haven't lost anything a few weeks down the line, it's worth using a calorie-counting website or book to double-check your calorie consumption on a typical Feast Day. As we saw in "The Math of Weight Loss" chapter, fasting will cut anything from 3,000 to 6,000 calories from your weekly consumption, but if you find you are bingeing or overcompensating, then the weight loss could be slow.

The good news is that most people find the Fast and Feast pattern helps them find a natural balance of enjoying food without overindulging. If someone had told me that at the beginning, I'd have been skeptical, but it really does happen.

It Gets Easier!

If you find your Fast Day tough, then take comfort from the fact that most of us have found they get easier—much easier. Many dieters look forward to Fast Days as they love the feeling of lightness and euphoria; feeling good physically, but also psychologically, knowing that you're doing something good for your body.

Reviewing and Planning Your Next Fasts

The first few weeks are about experimenting with what works for you—the best mealtimes, the most satisfying foods, plus trying to reduce any side effects you might feel.

Get into the habit of planning the days you'll be fasting the next week and preparing by buying ready meals or the ingredients for homemade dishes. Check the food section of this book for more ideas and options.

One thing to consider is whether you're someone who craves variety or a person who will be happy with the same foods on your Fast Day? I've mentioned my huge beet-fest that lasted for about a month during the diet without any side effects. Then gradually, and naturally, I switched to something else. If the idea of eating the same thing on Fast

Days will damage your motivation, then experiment and go onto forums to check out what ideas people have, especially for eating seasonally (which is also likely to be cheaper!).

Exercise and 5:2

Many people avoid vigorous exercise at first during Fast Days until they've discovered how their bodies react to the calorie restriction. I started going to the gym on Fast Days about a month after I began the diet. At first, I did feel light-headed at times and reduced the pace a little, but I've found that I can now keep up the same exercise intensity on Fast and Feast Days. One thing to note if you do exercise, don't eat extra on Fast Days to compensate for the calories burned.

> *I typically jog 6 kilometers [3.7 miles] four times a week. It makes no difference if that is a diet day.*
> *—Stephen, 47*

> *On fasting days I do thirty minutes on the treadmill at 2 mph. As I have arthritis at the moment, this is the most I can do without bringing on an "episode" of arthritis, but I hope to build it up as I lose weight/get fitter. I try to do this every day, but if I feel sore I will rest for a day or two.   —Sally, 49*

> *I haven't found it easy to exercise on Fast Days, but on other days I will spend two to three evenings a week*

in the gym doing weights, cardio, and swimming.
—Claire, 43

I've maintained my usual routine of daily exercise
(mostly cycling to work). I generally avoid tough
workouts on fasting days.   —James, 43

I run about four times a week, thirty [minutes] each
time. It doesn't really matter if I do it on Fast or non-
Fast Days because it doesn't increase my appetite. I
don't factor it into my calorie restriction because I don't
think it makes that much difference.   —Sarah, 37

There's a debate about whether exercising on Fast Days or on an empty stomach before breakfast, for example, might have benefits although an analysis on the British National Health Services website suggests that it's too early to draw conclusions (see links to this in the resources section). For now it's good to do what feels right for you, but do be wary of pushing yourself too hard at first, and consult your doctor if you have any doubts at all.

Weighing In

Most diets recommend weighing yourself no more than once a week because fluid levels and weight fluctuates so much, especially for women, during the monthly menstrual cycle. But Dr. Mosley has suggested daily weigh-ins as a tool for monitoring progress.

One of the first dieters in the Facebook group, Linda, has produced an amazing graph recording her weight every non-Fast day since she began, which she's kindly allowed me to reproduce. The bottom shows the passage of time and illustrates the variations graphically as well as showing the overall downward trend (we've kept the exact weights off—as Linda says, "A lady has to keep SOME secrets!").

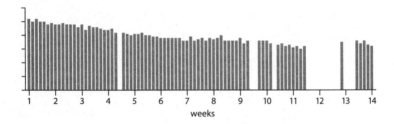

weeks

Linda explains how the graph has helped—and occasionally hindered—her.

There is quite a lot of variation from day to day. There are lots of reasons for the daily fluctuation: loss of water on fasting days due to depletion of stored glycogen; less gut content, fluid levels in the body, etc., as well as weight loss. In fact, fat loss will account for very little of the daily weight loss and is easily disguised by variations in stored glycogen and gut content. I also hit a period where food was going in but not much was coming out (to put it delicately) and there's a period there where I didn't fast because I had a cold and couldn't face it, and Xmas, of course.

Linda has fasted 32 times with a 500 calorie limit, which adds up to a calorie deficit overall of 48,000 calories, which should then equate to a loss of almost 14 pounds in total. In fact, she's lost more, possibly because her DCR is a bit higher than average, so potentially she could have eaten slightly more on Fast Days.

For her, (and for us!), keeping such a detailed record has been enlightening. But she also advises:

Please don't be despondent and give up if you weigh yourself after a fast or a week where you have been "good" and don't see as much of a loss as you might expect.

The risk of despondency is the reason I don't weigh myself every day. To me, it would be a roller coaster, even though I know there are good reasons for fluctuation. Sally feels the same:

> *I was tempted to weigh myself every day (and did!) when I started, but it can be a bit soul destroying as you'll find you'll lose weight on Fasting days then appear to put it back on again on Feasting days. It's best to weigh once a week.*   —Sally, 49

It may be a generalization, but I suspect that daily weigh-ins may suit men better, as they like to know where they are and may be less likely to have an emotional reaction!

> *If you can bear it, weigh every day, Fast and non-Fast, because you can track what's happening and the pattern of losing weight. Provided you stick to it, it'll still be downwards . . .*   —Kevin, 40

However often you decide to do it, record the figure in a notebook or on a weight loss website. I tend to weigh myself in the morning after the second Fast Day of a week, first thing, before I've eaten. At first it felt like cheating, but as long as you always do it at the same time, then your progress will become clear.

Rewarding Yourself

Any lifestyle change can be tricky, and it makes sense to find ways to reward yourself that don't involve food. The standard advice is to go for things like a long hot bath, a massage, new clothes.

But if you're not into girly (or manly) treats, or you haven't reached your goal weight, brainstorm other rewards: a new DVD box set or even a fitness DVD, a great novel, tickets for a show or a gallery, whatever you love doing that you don't always give yourself time to enjoy. You could put aside the money you're saving from your grocery bill to pay for the treats!

I have even been known to reward myself with a new recipe book for the days when I can enjoy cooking without feeling guilty. There's pleasure in the gloriously illogical knowledge that weight loss is contributing to my next delicious meal on a Feast Day!

The Gift of Food

I'd like to share one story from forty-three-year-old Jenny, who is finding that her fasts are making her see the world differently too.

It really is a very good way of eating (I don't call it a diet!) and have to say, on a vaguely hippie level, I feel humbled by the fact that I can choose to go hungry. A homeless girl stopped me in the street the other day and asked if I could spare her a pound for a hot drink. I've never been approached directly like that before. But something in my brain pinged and I realized that I had chosen not to nip out of the office for a [sandwich] and [can] of fruit since it was a fasting day. So I gave her the fiver I'd have spent on lunch. You'd think I'd given a wheelbarrow full of treasure. It's funny how things strike you at just the right time— homeless people are a factor in any big town or city, yet being approached by that girl seems like proper synchronicity. —Jenny, 43

Inspired by Jenny, I made a donation to a homelessness charity and will do the same when I hit weight loss milestones. If it's something that appeals to you, you might consider doing the same.

The Best Reward—It Works!

You should begin seeing the results of the diet itself pretty quickly—which is the biggest reward. Many of us see changes from week one. In January 2013, the Facebook group had members who'd lost six pounds in a week, while others haven't lost anything until the second or third weeks. My own weight loss was very undramatic but it felt sustainable and what kept me going was the knowledge that the health benefits were the most important thing to me.

Troubleshooting

Most people who embark on the diet find it sustainable and simple. But what if it's *not* working quite as well as you'd hoped?

- Review your Feast Days. Do a trial calorie count on one or two days. If it exceeds your DCR (daily calorific requirement; see the calculations in "Diet Calculations: How to Reach Your Goal" on page 97) by a large amount, you may need to adjust your portion sizes. The good thing about having fasted is that cutting back slightly should be very easy.

- There are a few people who stick to the diet but don't see the results. If you've done some calorie counting and you're not bingeing, it may be worth talking to your doctor about thyroid or other issues, especially if you've struggled on other diets before. Now move onto Part Three—it's all about the food!

PART THREE
EATING THE 5:2 WAY

Home Cooking or Ready-Made
Foods—You Choose!

Getting Started Eating the 5:2 Way

There's no point in lying about this: you can't eat much on your Fast Days. But even 500 to 600 calories can fill you up, and for most of us, it's far less daunting than a "true" fast where you'd eat nothing at all.

The way people structure their Fast Days varies—there's no right answer!

Usually have 100 grams [about 3.5 ounces] frozen fruit for breakfast (thawed, 29 calories). Weight Watchers tomato soup (76 calories) at lunchtime and either a Weight Watchers frozen meal in the evening, or fish or chicken with salad in the evening to make up to the 500, less if possible. Allow 60 calories for two coffees with milk during the day. Weight Watchers chicken and beef hotpots are about 230 calories each. —Steph, 49

1x coffee (with milk and sugar)
1x instant soup for lunch
2 pieces of fruit in late afternoon
A decent meal in the evening
Also drink herbal teas during the day if I feel peckish
—Sunil, 34

Shop-bought soups (as low-calorie as possible) and ready meals, with some veg and fruit. I aim for 500 calories and total it as I go.   —Val, 56

Oat So Simple Porridge with semi-skimmed [low-fat] milk at around 1 p.m. (180 calories); Batchelors Golden Vegetable Cup a Soup at around 4:30 p.m. (59 calories); dinner usually around 300 to 350 calories, often from the Hairy Bikers Diet Cookbook which is excellent as it doesn't include obvious "diet" dishes and gives calories per portion.   —Andrew, 42

I've started making dal, baked beans are good, salads are filling, make my own tomato soup with a half stock cube in a little boiling water, one-third tom puree added once that's dissolved, herbs and garlic puree added (the stuff in the tube), then topped up with more boiling water. Easy. I avoid hi-GI foods.   —Linda, 52

Yogurt, cuppa soup, and an omelet!   —Graeme, 38

As I outlined in Step Two, you will need to make decisions about how often you eat on your Fast Day—one, two, or three meals—and also whether you want to cook or use ready-made meals. Many of us do both, though as I carry on with this regimen I veer more toward spending the minimum time in the kitchen. I adore cooking but it's less fun when you're measuring every teaspoon of vinegar, or fretting over lemon juice.

In this part of the book, I make suggestions for ready-made *and* homemade options for breakfasts, lunches, and dinners, plus snacks and treats, as well as tips for eating out. Equally, if you want to munch on oats at snack time, or sip soup for breakfast, of course it's your call!

The recipes are pretty simple and do please adjust them as you wish. Or you can put your own dishes into the recipe section of the MyFitnessPal website to work out how many calories are in your favorite foods. You can make a huge batch of soup or stew and then measure it out into portions to freeze. This way you enjoy all the economic benefits of a homemade dish, but run less risk of accidentally going over the limit for the day.

I'm a vegetarian and I do recommend focusing on fruit and vegetables on your Fast Days as you'll get more for your calories—though there are meaty suggestions too.

Also bear in mind that some scientists say eating a lot of protein may switch on IGF-1, which may be counterproductive. Dr. Mosley has said he tries to stick to 2 ounces of protein on Fast Days (as an example, a medium egg contains approximately 7 grams protein, and 3.5 ounces of cooked chicken breast contains around 1 ounce protein). You may prefer to keep protein levels down—it's a balance, though, as protein contains more calories but tends to keep you full for longer.

I've also included an A to Z to give you new ideas for seasonal produce. Plus there's a list of sweet and savory snack ideas, for those times when you *need* something *now*!

Finally, I've included a section of daily menu ideas to help you get started, plus a template so you can plan your own meals.

Food and Fasting Tips

Measure, Measure, Measure (At Least Until You Get Used to It!)

Yes, measuring is a bit tedious but it can also be very enlightening—see more on how to measure in Part Two. It will really give you an insight into why we might be consuming more calories than we ever realized before. Weighing and then recording exactly what you're eating on the Fast Days— right down to a teaspoon of balsamic vinegar or a sprinkling of sunflower seeds—is the best way to avoid the temptation to cheat. Of course, once you're more used to the quantities you can eat on Fast Days, you won't need to measure so frequently.

Dollhouse Meals

The simplest approach to doing this diet is to cut out all snacks and then measure tiny portions of the foods you and your family normally eat (checking the calorie counts carefully until you can estimate them without looking at references). Sometimes it's easier than cooking something entirely separate when time is short. It helps to use smaller plates or dishes—I think of my Fast Day yogurt and fruit as a doll's house-sized portion.

Vitamin "Insurance"

It makes sense to take a multivitamin during the fasts, just to make sure you're getting enough nutrients. Of course, if you're eating lots of vegetables, you might be getting even higher levels of certain vitamins than usual, but I think taking a good multivitamin is a sensible move for anyone who is dieting.

Meal Replacement Shakes and Bars

There's no need to buy "special" foods for your Fast Days, and personally I prefer to eat foods that are similar to what I eat on normal days—just smaller portions or with fewer "naughty" additions.

Having said this, diet shakes, soups, and bars have proved useful for some people—they are fortified with vitamins and they also offer very precise calorie-controlled portions, so you know exactly what you're getting.

Although the milkshakes were boring, I can see the benefit and am pleased I took that route to start: A) I didn't have to think about calories on restricted days, therefore, I didn't think about food and B) because the milkshake was so restricting, choosing what to eat after the two weeks were up, has made me more aware of not to go over my calorie limit—and I don't want to.   —Anita, 51

I'd find them off-putting, but if you enjoy them or find them convenient, there's no reason why you shouldn't use them, so long as you eat a varied diet on Feast Days!

Savoring the Flavor

Unless you have chosen meal replacements, one good way to make your Fast Days more enjoyable is finding ways to add flavor without adding too many calories. This means that spices, fresh herbs, and lower-calorie sauces come into their own to add depth and keep your taste buds entertained. Take your pick from:

Chile: Red chile pepper flakes are excellent for pepping up soups, stews, and baked beans. One study also suggests they might help with fat-burning and increasing the metabolism. But go easy—they pack a punch. Fresh chiles are delicious too, but use them with even more caution.

Hot Chili Sauce: This is another easy way to liven things up. It contains more calories than chile flakes do, but you need very little.

Fresh Herbs: Herbs are a great addition to salad. The most versatile are chives and basil. Try chives with scrambled eggs or with other herbs in an omelet, basil torn up and added to tomato-based soups or stews/sauces. Though not strictly categorized as herbs, arugula or baby spinach can be used in small quantities to add their distinctive flavors to both salads and cooked dishes like soup or stews.

Garlic: Low in calories and a little goes a very long way. It's much less potent if you roast it along with other vegetables: break into cloves but leave them in their skins until they're roasted, then use as a puree. You can even spread on a slice of bread if you're brave; it's as unctuous as butter.

Horseradish/Wasabi: I love the scary-hot tang of wasabi (the green horseradish you get in pre-packed sushi trays or in a tube) even though the tiniest quantity is eye-watering. Great to take your mind off fasting, though!

Miso: This Japanese fermented paste comes in jars or tubes and adds a meaty (though it's vegetarian) flavor to all sorts of dishes, and also works as a very low-calorie soup stirred with boiling water in a mug. You can also buy it as powdered sachets ready to make into soup, which is more convenient to take to work.

Mustard: Like horseradish, it's hot and tasty and works with cheese, ham and other cold meats.

Relish/Chutney: I am addicted to all things sweet and sour, including relish and chutneys. Be mindful of the sugar content, but a small amount, calorie-counted, can give you a hit of flavor. Spread some very thinly on a slice of bread, add a slice of low-cal cheese, and grill for a Fast Day cheese on toast.

Salsa: Either buy fresh, in jars (still surprisingly tasty), or make your own (see the recipe under A to Z Ingredient Inspiration). It's great as an accompaniment to fish, lean meat, or Quorn/veggie burgers and as it contains no sugar, and it is a much better bet than tomato ketchup.

Soy Sauce: This is salty but definitely adds zing, as does Worcestershire sauce.

Vinegars: Cider or wine vinegars can work well as a dressing without oil, as can balsamic, though the latter is slightly more calorific as it's sweet, so measure it and count in your calorie allowance; it's around 16 calories per tablespoon. I also love tomatoes baked in the oven with a few drops of balsamic and then served with fresh herbs like basil or thyme.

What *Not* to Eat on Your Fast Day

Of course, you can eat what you like—up to your calorie limit—but here are some things that many people avoid on Fast Days:

Fruit and Fruit Juice

Juiced and many whole fruits may upset your blood sugar balance due to the natural sugars—you could be hit by cravings by 11 a.m. which is NOT what you want. The main exception is berries: strawberries, blueberries, and raspberries won't give you quite the same intense sugar hit, but they are strongly flavored. Frozen berries also work well when fresh aren't in season; blueberries and raspberries are particularly nice.

Refined Carbohydrates

White bread, potatoes, and white rice are particularly likely to give you that carb high that will then make you hungry "on the rebound." Complex carbohydrates—seeded rolls, brown rice, sweet potatoes—will have a less dramatic effect but you won't get a very big portion of these foods if you want to stay within your Fast Day calorie limit.

One approach to helping you find the foods that won't trigger sugar spikes, is the Glycemic Index, which measures how fast different foods are converted to sugar in the blood stream. It's not just the basic foods that vary; the variety and even the cooking method of something like potatoes has a dramatic effect. So boiled potatoes cause much less of a spike than a baked spud.

I've added some links about GI in the resources section. But remember, it's about finding what works for you. One 5:2 convert swears by a small baked potato as her main meal on a Fast Day!

Alcoholic Drinks

These are high in calories and won't fill you up. On an empty stomach, they could lower your willpower, too.

Confession time: I know it's nothing to be proud of, but I have been known to save 100 calories for a decent glass of wine if I am meeting friends after work. Obviously, you shouldn't be having 20 percent of your calories as alcohol on a regular basis, but wine—particularly brut sparkling wine—can be a very nice pick-me-up. Two glasses, though, and you probably won't be able to resist what everyone else is eating.

Breakfasts

For years, diet wisdom has been that breakfast is the most important meal of the day, but I'm one of many 5:2 Dieters to discover that I don't actually need it. In fact, on Fast Days, many people seem to find that the longer they can delay their first meal, the less hungry they feel. However, if you can't face the day without it, there are lots of options for you.

Ready-Made Options

With ready-made breakfasts, it makes sense to get label-savvy. Many cereals are so high in sugar that they could really knock you off course.

Cereals

Many 5:2 dieters avoid sweetened packaged cereals due to the blood sugar highs and lows they cause. Also, the portions when you measure them out are really tiny. Oatmeal or bran cereals are probably a better bet, or some low-sugar mueslis or granolas, including several mainstream brands—look for higher fiber and lower carbohydrate counts on the label.

Cereal Bars

These are marketed as healthy alternatives to normal cereals, but have many of the same drawbacks. Many come in at 100 calories or so but are so sweet you'll be craving another one within an hour or less. I used to love one particular brand but always ended up eating two, which defeated the purpose, because I could have had a normal snack instead for fewer calories! A product test of cereal bars in the UK, for example, showed that one contained almost 4 teaspoons' worth of sugar.

Oatmeal

Nutritionists often recommend oats as a good breakfast cereal because they release energy in the body slowly. For portion control, a premeasured packet like Quaker Instant Oatmeal works well for some dieters. However, choose versions with no added sugar. It's better to make it with water to save calories, but if you can't bear it, low-fat milk will still keep the calories under 200.

Smoothies

Pure fruit smoothies might seem tempting for a meal on the go, but they are not ideal, for the reasons given in the previous chapter: fruit can wreak havoc with blood sugar and make you hungry very fast. But those smoothies with yogurt, oats, and other slowly digested ingredients may be a better bet. Look at the calorie counts but also at the sugar/carbohydrate count on the label—the lower the better.

Yogurt

There are so many varieties of yogurt that you need to be label savvy. I love the richness of Greek yogurt and prefer having a tiny portion of that on a Fast Day to more of a low-fat variety. As always, follow your taste buds. A good breakfast option can be a natural low-fat, low-carb yogurt that you add a few nuts or seeds to (again, measured carefully) to stave off hunger pangs later. Sunflower or pumpkin seeds will work, along with a few fresh seasonal strawberries or frozen raspberries or blueberries.

Homemade Breakfasts

Something on Toast

Who can resist toast? It's the crack cocaine of the carbohydrate world for me, so it can be a risky choice on a Fast Day. But if you can stick to one or two slices without butter, it can make your mornings more bearable. Be sure to check labels carefully as a slice of bread could vary from 80 calories for smaller slices all the way up to over 150!

The following are for the topping only and I've used a range of different brands—most supermarkets will have similar products:

FOOD	CALORIES
Medium poached egg, 1	75–85
Heinz Snap Pot Baked Beans, 200g	144
Heinz Home Style Beans (Chipotle BBQ Style), ½ cup	130
Skippy Natural Creamy Peanut Butter, 1 teaspoon	31
Philadelphia Extra Light Cream Cheese, .3 ounces	11
Deli sliced boiled ham, 1 slice	80
Kraft Singles American Cheese Slices, 1 slice	60

Go to Work on Just an Egg?

Eggs are protein-rich, but they can also be very satisfying, especially at breakfast, so they're worth considering. Poaching or boiling are the lowest-calorie ways of preparing eggs, but they can also be fried using oil sprays, which typically work out to 1 calorie per spray. They're not as tasty as butter, but they won't eat up your entire calorie allowance either.

Breakfast Recipes

Basic Scrambled Eggs
(155 calories)

I know most of us have our own ways of making scrambled eggs, but here's one that always works:

Take 2 large eggs (approx. 70 calories each), crack into a mug or cup, and add 2 tablespoons of semi-skimmed milk (about 15 calories). Beat well with a fork until the yolks and whites are combined. Season with salt and pepper.

Spray a small nonstick saucepan with low- or no-calorie nonstick spray and set over low to medium heat. The more slowly you cook the eggs, the less rubbery they'll be. Add egg mixture and cook for 1 minute without stirring.

Then begin to move the eggs around the pan with a spoon or spatula, until the eggs begin to set or thicken, depending on how you prefer them. Cook thoroughly if you are making this for someone who is pregnant or immune-compromised. Remember that the mixture will keep heating as long as it's in the hot pan, so serve immediately.

ADDITIONS:
Fresh herbs, chopped
Chile flakes
Mushrooms, cooked in no-calorie spray
Chopped ham or smoked salmon (a little goes a long way)

SERVING SUGGESTION: Instead of serving on toast, use no-calorie nonstick spray to fry large portobello mushrooms for 4 to 5 minutes (turning halfway) and top with the eggs.

Anytime Omelets
(140 calories)

I'm a fan of omelets because to me they seem more complete without the addition of the (calorific) toast.

Break 2 large eggs (about 70 calories each) into a bowl and whisk well until combined. Season with salt and pepper.

Use a small nonstick frying or omelet pan and no- or low-calorie nonstick spray, and heat the pan until it's hot but not burning: apparently you should be able to touch it with the back of your hand but I would caution against doing this!

Add the egg and keep the mix moving for 1 to 2 minutes so that all the uncooked egg has contact with the pan.

Then hold the pan at an angle and let the omelet move towards the site of the pan; use a spatula to fold a third of the omelet back on itself. Do it again for the other side until it's a cigar shape.

Again, you can add extras, either to the center of the omelet when it's partially cooked but before the fold, or to the basic egg mixture.

Homemade Oatmeal

There are many different brands available, so pick your favorite.
Use instant oats for the fastest result—each brand will have
microwave or stovetop cooking instructions on the package.

Basic Bircher Muesli
(185 calories)

This is how I like my oats. I first discovered it on vacation in the
upscale hotel buffet, and it's filling and healthy. It was invented
by the Swiss physician Maximilian Bircher-Benner to help
his patients improve their health through diet. It's also almost
effortless and tastes a lot yummier than it sounds. The only
problem is that it makes a very small (but very filling!) portion in
a bowl, but I'm getting used to those dollhouse-sized servings.

Mix 1 ounce porridge oats (116 calories) with 1½
tablespoon of 1 percent milk (10 calories) or apple juice
(11 calories) in a bowl or plastic container. Store in the
fridge overnight, covered.

In the morning, if it's a little bit dry, add slightly more
liquid. Grate half a small apple over the top (27 calories),
mix in, and add 2 tablespoons of plain low-fat yogurt (17
calories) plus any of the ingredients suggested below for
porridge—berries are especially good.

Take it to work in a Tupperware!

THINGS TO ADD TO OATMEAL

FOOD	CALORIES
1 teaspoon honey	20
1 teaspoon sunflower seeds	30
1 teaspoon golden raisins	15
½ grated very small apple (approx. 1 ounce)	27
20 raspberries (frozen are fine: add them to unheated oats straight from the freezer before cooking when fresh berries aren't available)	20 (1 calorie each!)
50 blueberries	39
1 tablespoon low-fat yogurt	Check label!
1 tablespoon unsweetened cocoa powder	12
1 teaspoon powdered cinnamon (a teaspoon may be too much!)	6

Cool Lunches, Hot Dinners

Again, I've split this into ready-made meals that other dieters and I have found filling and tasty, and then suggestions for homemade dishes. You can obviously have them for lunch, dinner, or even breakfast, if you feel like it. It's your diet.

Ready-Made Options

Frozen Main Dishes

If you choose to eat one main meal a day, then it will be really easy to find ready-made meals that come in at 500 to 600 calories a serving. Try to choose menus with a balance of protein and carbohydrates to keep you from getting hungry again too quickly (a chocolate cheesecake or brownie dessert might come in under the limit but will probably drive you crazy with hunger again within a couple of hours).

The following frozen dishes are lower in calories than traditional versions of the same dishes; be sure to read the labels for salt and other additives.

Lean Cuisine: Lean Cuisine (leancuisine.com) has a vast set of choices, including the "spa collection" and over ninety products without preservatives, including Grilled Chicken Primavera at 220 calories or Hunan Stir-Fry with Beef at 280 calories. Read the reviews to find out which ones dieters enjoy the most!

Smart Ones from Weight Watchers: Smart Ones from Weight Watchers (eatyourbest.com) include Satisfying Selections that are designed to keep you full with extra protein. It includes Peppercorn Beef at 280 calories. There's also a star rating system on the website so you can see what other people have liked—the Chicken in Spicy Peanut Sauce gets a high rating, and is 250 calories.

Healthy Choice: Healthy Choice (healthychoice.com) offers a range of vegetarian options that are free of additives and include dishes like Pumpkin Squash Ravioli at 310 calories. The Cafe Steamers get the thumbs up, especially the Honey Glazed Turkey and Sweet Potatoes at 250 calories. Lots of reviews on this site too.

Kashi: Kashi's frozen meals (kashi.com) are less widely available but have an emphasis on whole grains in dishes like Sesame Chicken and Pilaf at 300 calories.

Amy's Kitchen: Amy's Kitchen (amys.com) also has its fans, with lots of vegetarian and gluten-free options. The Cheese Enchilada is gluten free and has only 240 calories.

Soups

Making your own soup is easy and cheap, but for a no-hassle option, I often buy ready-made and the flavors and brands keep on improving (they used to taste very salty but I find the newer versions less heavy handed). It's a great option in colder weather when a salad, however low in calories, doesn't quite seem to fill you up. There's also scientific evidence that eating soup keeps you fuller, because it stays in the stomach for longer.

The fresh soups market doesn't exist in the same way in the U.S. as it does for me in the UK, but there are still plenty of options.

Wal-Mart Marketside: The Wal-Mart Marketside collection includes a number of "fresh" soup options without additives in microwaveable containers. It includes a Vegetable Soup at 90 calories per serving and Chicken Vegetable Pasta at 100 calories per serving.

Campbell's: Campbell's (campbellsoup.com) has an extensive selection of soups, including a Healthy Request collection with dishes like Mexican-Style Chicken Tortilla Soup at 110 calories per portion, and many of them are available in microwave packs to take to work.

There's also Campbell's **GO range,** which has chunkier soups served in pouches, like the Spicy Chorizo & Pulled Chicken with Black Beans at 210 calories for the pack.

I often eat a portion of soup for lunch and dinner with a small slice of bread (I noticed when I tried to eat only soup, I missed the texture of other foods as much as the calories). Again, I like the convenience of having my day's meals in a single container—great for work.

Grains and Noodles

Pasta won't offer you much bulk for your calories, but if you want something more solid than soup and just as convenient, you could look at the microwaveable rice pouches that have extra flavors and spices built in. One of these will probably add up to around 400 calories for the packet, so serve it in two portions, perhaps with some frozen vegetables added. I'd definitely try to choose the brown rice versions as white rice will usually make you hungry again much faster. Uncle Ben's Spanish Style, for example, at 200 calories for half a pack is a great option.

We're moving toward homemade in this category, but there's been a lot of talk on diet forums lately about "no-calorie" shirataki noodles, which are made of a kind of yam and are supposed to leave you full but not add to your calorie count. They're so popular they've been sold out wherever I go, but I've heard mixed reports. Yes, they're filling, and they can work well combined with a stir-fry or some prawns or lean meat. However, don't expect them to taste too much like "real" noodles. They can also have a slightly fishy smell so if you do use them, rinse them well before cooking.

Preparing couscous could count as borderline cooking, but there are various flavored couscous brands that you put in a bowl and simply add boiling water to. Again, you can bulk them out with frozen peas or corn, or serve with a veggie sausage or burger.

Homemade Main Dishes

All the egg dishes and "on toast" dishes from the Breakfast chapter will work equally well at another time of day: poached egg on toast is one of those dishes you can eat without anyone really noticing you're on a diet.

In this section, I'll stick to simple dishes that barely count as recipes. They're more suggestions for fast and easy meals when you don't want to spend too much time cooking or in reach of temptations.

A Good, Square Meal

You obviously need to be a little more careful about your meat and vegetable meals while you're fasting, but it certainly doesn't mean giving them up!

I've created a mix and match table with some suggestions for combinations and portion size: treat all the calorie counts as a guideline and double check on the back of your packs. Most steamed and boiled green veggies come in at around 30 to 35 calories per 3.5 ounces, though peas and corn are higher in calories.

MEAT/FISH	VEG 1	VEG 2	TOTAL CALORIES
Salmon 1 small steak, 3.5 ounces, 135 calories	Mange tout/ snow peas 100g, 32 calories	Mushrooms fried in no-calorie spray 2 ounces, 10 calories	177
Tuna 1 steak 2.5 ounces, 115 calories	Sweet corn 2.5 ounces canned, 50 calories	Spinach ½ cup cooked & drained, 32 calories	197
Prawns 3.5 ounces, 80 calories	Roast tomatoes 10 cherry tomatoes 30 calories roasted with no calorie spray & 1 teaspoon balsamic, 5 calories	Green beans 3.5 ounces, approx. 30 calories	145
Chicken 3.5 ounces breast fillet, 100–140 calories	Broccoli 1 cup, steamed 30 calories	Sliced mixed peppers 3 ounces, 25 calories	155–195
Turkey 3.5 ounces breast fillet, 100–140 calories	Baby carrots frozen 3 ounces, 18 calories	Cauliflower 100g steamed, 25 calories	143–183
Quorn burger 1.75 ounces, 80 calories	Sweet potato (small: 133g), 105 calories	Garden peas 50, 34 calories	219

Cool Lunches and Hot Dinners Recipes

The recipes that follow are simple, fresh, and infinitely adaptable. Use them as the basis for healthy, nutritious, low-calorie meals on Fast Days.

For any meal, vegetables make ideal "vessels" for other ingredients. They're low in calories but colorful and tasty for Fast Days! Portobello mushrooms are large and flat, as big as hamburgers, and make wonderful containers for fillings. I tend to grill or microwave them with the fillings. They're so low in calories that you could also serve them as "burgers" if they've been grilled or fried in no-calorie nonstick spray!

Easy Vegetable Curry
(150 calories per serving; makes 2)

Replace the vegetables with any others in season, being sure to adjust the calories, of course. Also, you can serve with a portion of meat or fish. As a guideline, use the portion sizes and calorie counts listed in the table above. Grill or bake the meat or fish and either chop into smaller pieces and add to the curry mix, or serve with the curry as a side dish.

1 teaspoon oil

2 cloves garlic, crushed

1 medium onion, finely chopped

1 teaspoon chili powder

1 teaspoon ground ginger

1 teaspoon ground turmeric

3½ ounces green beans, sliced

7 ounces cauliflower or broccoli, broken into small florets

3½ ounces carrots, sliced

3½ ounces potatoes, diced

1 teaspoon tomato puree

1½ tablespoons golden raisins

Warm the oil in a large pan, add the garlic and onion, and cook for 5 minutes. Add the spices and cook gently for 1 minute more. Add all the vegetables and 1¼ cups (300 ml) of water, then add the other ingredients. Heat until the water boils, then reduce the heat and cover; cook for about 30 minutes. This keeps well in the fridge for 48 hours if you want to save till your next Fast Day.

Mediterranean Roasted Vegetables
(148 calories per serving; makes 4)

This is good with whatever herbs or spices you like; try chile flakes. Mushrooms, baby corn, or slices of butternut squash (in ½-inch/1-cm slices so they bake through) taste great too. If you make more than you need, make soup: add to a large saucepan with water and a can of tomatoes, and bring to a boil. Adjust the water to make the consistency you like. When it's cooled down, blend in the pan with a stick (immersion) blender.

3 tablespoons olive oil

4 large zucchini, sliced

5 plum tomatoes, sliced

2 eggplants, sliced

1 large garlic bulb (don't peel)

A bunch of rosemary, broken into sprigs, or oregano or thyme

salt and pepper

Preheat the oven to 425°F (220°C). Drizzle 1 tablespoon of the oil into a baking pan or ovenproof dish, then layer the vegetables across the dish with the garlic head in the middle. Poke the herbs in among the layered vegetables, add 1 tablespoon of olive oil over the top and season with salt and pepper.

Roast for 45 minutes to 1 hour until the vegetables are charred around the edges, adding the remaining oil during cooking. (You can use less oil, but it's already a very small, healthy amount!)

Serve with the still-wrapped cloves of garlic, to be squeezed out over the vegetables.

So-Easy Stir-Fry

(160 calories per serving; makes 2 very generous servings)

This is another basic recipe that you can adapt with different vegetables; peppers and scallions would be nice. Or buy stir-fry veggie packs from the grocery store.

If you want to use meat or fish, pre-fry these in the oil to make sure they're cooked through. Then set aside, fry the veggies in the same pan, and heat through all the ingredients after adding the soy and chili sauce. For vegetarian protein, just after you add the soy and chili sauce, add thinly sliced tofu or a beaten egg.

1 tablespoon vegetable oil

1 red chile, sliced (omit for less heat)

1 garlic clove, sliced

1 pound mixed vegetables such as bok choy, baby corn, and broccoli

1 ½ tablespoons soy sauce

2 tablespoons sweet chili sauce

Heat the oil in a wok or frying pan, then fry the chile, if using, and garlic for 1 minute. Add the vegetables and make sure they've all been coated in oil. Fry for 2 to 3 minutes, then add the soy and chili sauces and cook for another 2 to 3 minutes until the vegetables are tender.

Spicy Indian Lentil & Tomato Soup
(130 calories per serving; makes 2)

A very simple, warming soup made from the things you have in your pantry. Double the portions and freeze the extra, if you like.

1 onion, chopped

pinch of red chile pepper flakes

2 tablespoons red lentils

1 (14-ounce) can chopped tomatoes

2 cups vegetable stock

½ bunch cilantro, or to taste

salt and pepper

Put all the ingredients, except the cilantro, in a pan together and heat until simmering. Cover and cook for 20 minutes until the lentils are soft, then add the cilantro, cook for 1 minute, and blend with a stick (immersion) blender. Season with salt and pepper, and serve.

Mushroom Tom Yum Soup

(40 calories per serving; makes 4 servings)

Very tasty, very fast and very low in calories.

4¼ cups chicken or vegetable stock

1 to 2 tablespoons tom yum paste

7 ounces fresh mushrooms (ideally a mixture including oyster and shiitake)

4 dried shiitake mushrooms rehydrated in water (remove any hard edges)

juice of 1 lime

1 tablespoon fish sauce, or to taste

1 sliced red chile pepper

cilantro, to taste

Bring the stock to the boil in a large pan. Add the tom yum paste and then the mushrooms. Simmer for 5 minutes before adding the other ingredients. Season and add more fish sauce as needed before serving.

Green and White Super Soup

(76 calories per serving; makes 2 servings)

Super-vitamins, super-easy.

½ bunch green onions, chopped

1 teaspoon olive oil

1 small potato, peeled and diced

2 cups vegetable stock

5 ounces mixed watercress, spinach, and arugula

salt and pepper

Cook the green onions in the olive oil until soft. Add the potato and cook for 2 more minutes, then add the stock and simmer until the potato is tender, 10 to 15 minutes depending on the size of the dice. Add the greens, simmer for 1 minute, and then use a stick (immersion) blender to blend till smooth. Season with salt and pepper, and serve.

Almost-Instant Corn Chowder

(115 calories; makes 1 serving)

1 medium green onion

1½ cups vegetable stock

3½ ounces frozen sweet corn

pinch of red chile pepper flakes

4 teaspoons low-fat milk

salt and pepper

In a medium pan, fry the onion in no-calorie nonstick spray. Add all the ingredients except the milk, simmer for 5 minutes, then add the milk and blend lightly with a stick (immersion) blender. Season with salt and pepper, and serve.

Philly Mushrooms
(66 calories for 2)

Take 2 large, flat mushrooms (about 4.5 ounces, 20 calories) and wipe with a kitchen towel. Spoon 2 tablespoons light cream cheese with herbs or chives (such as Philadelphia brand) into the mushrooms and top with chopped herbs or black pepper: either grill for 2 minutes until heated through or microwave for 30 to 45 seconds.

The Mediterranean filling for the stuffed avocado recipe below also works well in mushrooms or peppers.

Stuffed Avocado
(125 calories, plus your choice of filling)

Avocados are high in fat but filling and tasty. You can serve them cold, of course, but also hot if you want to try something different. Their shape makes a nice "bowl" for all sorts of fillings. Use half a medium Hass avocado (125 calories; save the other half in the fridge to use later the same day—store with the stone still inside and a little lemon juice on the cut surface to stop it discoloring) and add whatever fillings you like:

Guacamole-style: Add store-bought salsa, or a mix of 2 chopped cherry tomatoes, a sprinkle of red chile pepper flakes, and half a chopped medium green onion (less than 10 calories).

Cream cheese–style: Add 1 tablespoon light cream cheese, any flavor (20 calories). This can be microwaved for 20 to 30 seconds or grilled for about 5 minutes to serve as a kind of pâté with whole-grain crackers. Spray first with no-calorie cooking spray before grilling.

Arugula and balsamic vinegar: Pour 1 tablespoon (15 calories) balsamic vinegar into the hollow of the avocado, add a good handful of arugula leaves (.75 ounce, or, is a lot and just 4 calories) and grind plenty of pepper and sea salt on top.

Prawns and lime: Fill the hollow with 2 ounces of cooked prawns (about 45 calories) plus the juice of half a lime (under 10 calories) to serve. Or use low-cal dressing of your choice in place of the lime juice.

Mediterranean hot: Spray the avocado with no-calorie cooking spray and grill for 5 minutes or microwave for 20 to 30 seconds. In the hollow, place a mixture of 1 chopped sun-dried tomato with the oil drained off, 2 pitted olives, a few capers, ½ a green onion, and some torn basil or arugula leaves (filling is less than 20 calories).

Quickest-Ever Stuffed Pepper
(92 calories for 2 halves)

Halve a medium red or yellow bell pepper (31 calories) and pull out the core and ribs. Add three cherry tomatoes to each half (18 calories for 6 tomatoes) and a sliced medium green onion (5 calories). Top with 2 tablespoons light cream cheese (any savory flavor, 40 calories) plus other flavorings from suggestions in "Savoring the Flavor" on page 140.

Grill for 10 to 12 minutes or roast in oven at 400°F (200°C) for around 30 minutes, until the pepper flesh is soft and the edges are charred.

Salads

A prewashed bag of lettuce contains very few calories and is a canvas for a great Fast Day salad.

SALAD INGREDIENT	CALORIES
½ bag pre-washed salad—whichever you like!	15–30; see label
Cherry tomatoes	3 per tomato
Sliced bell pepper	30 per pepper
Beetroot, 1.75 ounces cooked	16
Sweet corn—1.75 ounces drained from tin	40–50
Spring onion / scallion: medium	8
Parmesan—great shaved thinly with potato slicer	10g shavings 40
Cottage cheese: varies depending on fat content	60–100 per 100g
Wafer thin ham (deli style)—slice varies	10–15 per slice
Wafer thin turkey (deli style)—slice varies	8–15 per slice
Cooked prawns	50g = 40
Smoked salmon—1 2-ounce slice	80–100
Artichoke hearts: depends on size of can	25–50 per portion
Pumpkin seeds: 1 teaspoon	29
Pine nuts: 1 teaspoon	35
Sunflower seeds: 1 teaspoon	30
Buffalo mozzarella, ½ container (2.2 ounces)	170
Chopped apple: ½ small apple (approx. 1.75 ounces)	27
Walnuts: 1 teaspoon	34
Whole boiled egg	70–80

A to Z Ingredient Inspiration

This chapter is designed to give you a little boost if you're bored and are looking for quick new ideas.

FOOD	IDEAS	CALORIES
A is for Asparagus	Super-nutritious, filling, and delicious, either steamed, boiled, or—easiest of all—microwaved. Serve with sea salt and pepper, lemon juice, or a nice poached egg on the side to dip into! You can also precook and then grill. It's a great summer dish.	5 spears = 25 calories
A is also for Almonds	These are so good, and although like all nuts they're calorific, a small handful can be very filling. I've also used them ground—a teaspoon mixed with yogurt and berries gives you a hint of sweetness while containing negligible carbs, so you'll stave off the hunger pangs for longer.	1 whole = 7 calories 1 teaspoon = 31 calories

FOOD	IDEAS	CALORIES
B is for Beets	You might have gathered that I am a bit of a beet fiend, especially for those that have been flavored with chili or baked with ground cumin and served with a little low-fat yogurt. Beets are very good for you, and make a delicious salad with arugula, cherry tomatoes, balsamic vinegar, and chopped fresh apple. I also like beets with fresh mozzarella (the kind that comes floating in water).	1.75 ounces cooked = 16 calories
B is also for Broccoli	Another one of those super-foods you hear about, broccoli is horrible when it's overcooked, but steaming it works well. Or have you tried frying until it almost turns black? The edges caramelize if you slice through the florets into ¼-inch pieces, then heat some spray oil in a pan until very hot, and fry on both sides. You need the kitchen fan for this one or an open window as it can smoke, but it's great with pepper and sea salt, soy sauce, or chili sauce, and is very low in calories.	3.5 ounces = 38 calories
C is for Chocolate	You can't have too much of it, but two or four squares of the dark, expensive kind can be enough to satisfy a craving. It's sweet, but not too sweet, and high in antioxidants.	4 small squares (.3 ounces) = 58 calories
D is for Dijon mustard	I add Dijon (or really any kind of mustard) to lots of savory dishes to give a low-calorie kick. There are calories in mustard, but it's so hot that you only need a little.	1 teaspoon = 15 calories
E is for Edamame	Those whole pods that are served in Asian restaurants are available frozen to eat at home, and they're filling, nutritious, and can satisfy a snack craving.	1.75 ounces = 61 calories

The 5:2 Diet

FOOD	IDEAS	CALORIES
F is for low-fat Feta cheese	This cheese has a strong, salty taste, so a little goes a long way. Try it in a Greek salad with lots of tomato, black olives, and cucumber, and perhaps with some red wine vinegar or a premade lower-calorie dressing.	1.75 ounces = 100–120 calories
G is for Ginger	One of your best friends for extra flavor during Fast Days. I'm a big fan of the clean taste of the pickled ginger that's served with sushi—I'm addicted to it on its own!	.75 ounces (plenty!) = 10–15 calories
H is for Ham	Great for when you're having a savory craving. Prosciutto is fancy—try 2 slices of Prosciutto ham with 6 thin slices of melon.	Ham and melon = 80 calories
I is for Ice Cream (and frozen yogurt)	They don't have to be out of bounds if you choose carefully. Look for Italian-style ice cream, which is typically less fatty than American-style, or a creamy low-fat frozen yogurt (check the calories though, as some can be even higher than normal ice cream).	Varies by brand; be sure to read labels
J is for Jell-O	Sugar-free Jell-O can help overcome a sweet craving with negligible calories. Either buy ready-made or make up dishes in your own favorite flavor.	3–10 calories for a 3-ounce ready-made snack cup
K is for Kiwi	Often overlooked, maybe because of their unpromising exteriors, kiwis have a frenzy of vitamin C inside.	40 calories for a single small fruit
L is for Lentils	Cheap red lentils make a great base for soup (page "Spicy Indian Lentil & Tomato Soup" on page 83) and the "gourmet" French green variety are extremely filling and provide a nutritious and tasty base for a salad.	3.5 ounces ready-to-eat French green lentils = 130 calories

FOOD	IDEAS	CALORIES
M is for Mint	Mint is fantastic for digestion, and even people who dislike other herb teas often enjoy a mint infusion. It's so easy to grow and also makes a delicious addition to sparkling water. Add a crushed lime segment and you've got what I call a "nojito"!	Fewer than 5 calories for a huge handful
N is for Noodles	Try the shirataki "no-calorie" noodles, which can be found in the refrigerated section of your grocer and contain fewer than 20 calories per serving (and sometimes none at all). The ones with tofu taste less "fishy" and it's best to use a strong-flavored sauce and also to "dry roast" them for a minute in a hot pan before using!	Fewer than 20 calories per serving
O is for Oreo Cookies	Maybe it's because they look so cute, but I adore Oreos, and the mini versions can give you a sweet hit without too many calories if you can stop at one or two.	4 bite-size cookies = 65 calories
P is for Popsicles	Make your own low-cal ice pops with sugar-free squash, diluted fruit juice, low-fat yogurt, or pureed fruit. Freeze in a reusable mold and go wild!	Varies by fillings
Q is for Quinoa	Quinoa (pronounced "keen-wah") is a seed originally grown by the Incas that is used as a grain in pilafs or as a stuffing. It's very high in protein, so a little will fill you up and you can use it in salads or other dishes that are normally made with rice.	3.5 ounces cooked = 100–110 calories
R is for Ricotta	A lovely light Italian cheese with a mousse-like texture perfect for dips, sauces, or even as a substitute for mayonnaise in salads that need "binding." Check labels to get lower calorie versions.	1 cup = 50–100 calories, depending on brand

FOOD	IDEAS	CALORIES
S is for Salsa	The store-bought stuff can be really good, but nothing beats homemade. This one improves after a day in the fridge: soak 1 finely chopped medium onion in 2 tablespoons vinegar and 1 tablespoon salt overnight. Roast a medium red bell pepper until the skin is charred, discard the seeds and ribs, and chop the flesh. Add to the onion along with 1 finely diced tomato, ½ finely diced cucumber, and ½ finely diced celery stick. Stir in 1 more tablespoon salt, 1 teaspoon Worcestershire, and a pinch each of red chile pepper flakes, black pepper, and oregano. Makes 8 servings.	1 serving = 14 calories
T is for Turkey (and Thanksgiving)	Turkey is a great low-fat meat, but the rest of the celebration dishes are not that Fast Day–friendly, so I'd use the flexibility of this diet to eat what you like on the holiday itself, and then cut back later. It's a Feast Day, after all.	
T is for Tangerine	Easy to peel and the perfect portion size. Tangerines are also one of the newest super-foods, with research suggesting a chemical in the fruit can reduce the risk of heart attacks, diabetes, and stroke, as well as staving off obesity.	1 small tangerine = 37 calories
U is for Ugli fruit	This is a tough letter! I've never had an ugli. Apparently it's a bit like a grapefruit.	½ fruit = 45 calories

FOOD	IDEAS	CALORIES
V is for Vinegar	Vinegar is under-rated. The world of vinegar includes fruit vinegars, sherry, cider, red, and white wine and even champagne—and these are virtually calorie free. As a dressing, the milder ones can work on their own, without oil, and balsamic, which does contain more calories than some others, is fabulous on cooked vegetables, as well as salad. Plus apparently it has lots of medicinal benefits, including positive effects on blood pressure, cholesterol, and diabetes/insulin sensitivity.	1 teaspoon balsamic vinegar = 12–16 calories 1 teaspoon white wine vinegar = 1 calorie!
W is for Watercress	Watercress is another one of those ingredients often quoted as a super-food because of its high levels of vitamin C and other nutrients; it was recommended in the sixteenth century as a treatment for scurvy. It makes a nutritious salad or soup ingredient, and scientists are investigating its cancer-fighting properties too.	3.5 ounces = 11 calories
X is for Xmas	As with Thanksgiving, the treats like spiral ham and cheesecake won't help with Fast Days. But this diet is ideal for any kind of celebration. You can feel virtuous by simply fasting two days over the festive period, which might be a relief after so much rich food. Remember, this is for life, not just for Christmas.	

The 5:2 Diet

FOOD	IDEAS	CALORIES
Y is for Yogurt	Remember the thin, unpleasant-smelling diet yogurts of the eighties and nineties? Now you can get very palatable tasting ones at fewer than 100 calories. On Fast Days, though, I often prefer to use normal yogurt or even Greek yogurt in very tiny dollhouse portions.	Varies by brand
Z is for Zucchini	These summery vegetables are delicious stuffed or cooked on a griddle. Or use them as a lower-calorie substitute for pasta: slice into the thinnest "noodles" possible and blanch/boil in salted water for just one minute before serving with your favorite pasta sauce.	1 medium zucchini = 33 calories

Treats, Snacks, and Eating Out

To Snack or Not to Snack

The debate about "grazing" or snacking is one we've touched on in the book, and generally many 5:2 dieters do avoid eating between (small) meals on Fast Days. But there are times when you just want something NOW, and then it makes sense to go for the lower-calorie options rather than choose something that will undo the good you've done by fasting.

Health food stores are a good source of nuts or trail mix, but do check the nutritional values. My favorite snack food ever—Thai chili rice crackers—look as though they should be super-healthy but most are very high in calories.

I'm a fan of the company Graze.com, which delivers snacks in a letter-box sized container, with four mini-packs of sweet and savory snacks including nuts, dried fruit, and even chocolate mixes. Some are healthier than others, but opening the pack every week is like getting a little present.

The 5:2 Diet

You can ask for a light option, and they usually offer the first boxes at half-price.

I tend to find I crave either something sweet or savory, so here are some options for those moments when a mug of green tea won't do.

Savory Snacks and Treats

SNACK	CALORIES
Miso soup: most packets of miso soup with tofu or sea vegetables	25–35
Air popped popcorn, 1 cup	31
Olives: 10 pitted green olives	42
Rice cake Plus 2 teaspoons light cream cheese Or 1 teaspoon peanut butter as a topping	35–50 15 30
10 almonds (1 almond is 7 calories—will fill you up for ages)	70
1 strip of grilled bacon	45
10 Pringles	100

Sweet Snacks and Treats

SNACK	CALORIES
Sugar-free Jell-O snack cup	5–15
1 packet Swiss Miss diet hot chocolate	26
Milky Way Mini	40

SNACK	CALORIES
Small scoop of soft-scoop vanilla ice-cream	50–60
1 square (.3 ounces) 85 percent dark chocolate	55
2 medium peaches	76
20 cherries	80
1 small banana	90
5 dried apricots	95
4 dates	96

Eating Out

I am veering into the department of the obvious here, but I try not to eat out on Fast Days as it's really hard to make good choices, plus you have no real idea how many calories you're consuming. You will have read earlier on in my diary about when I went out planning to have soup at my favorite cafe, only to find it's not served on weekends. So I sprung for eggs Florentine, which was probably my entire daily allowance, but kept me full all day.

If you're out and about, make the choices you'd make for other diets—ask for bread to be taken off the table, or give it to your dining companion. Choose soups, ideally non-creamy, and salads, and ask for the dressing on the side. Lean fish or chicken with veggies is not exciting but will usually give you some control. If all else fails—if you want to give into temptation or suddenly have something to celebrate—then it's even simpler. Fast tomorrow instead!

Fast Day Meal Plans for All Tastes

You've got all the tools you need to plan your own Fast Days, but as an extra aid, I've outlined some daily meal plans using the recipes in this book and ready-made meals. Use them as the basis for your own meal planning if you find it useful, or go your own way! There's also a blank template for your own use.

Of course, men get an extra 100 calories on top of the 500 allowed for women, so I've added an extra Man's Ration to those days!

A page number after the dish means the recipe is in this book.

The Big Salad Lunch Day

This is one of my real-meal Fast Days: a massive, delicious, no-holds-barred salad eaten outdoors with friends on a picnic. Slightly over in terms of calories, but plenty of protein and fat that keeps me from getting hungry until the next day.

MEAL	FOOD	CALORIES
Breakfast		
Lunch	Buffalo mozzarella, 2.2 ounces	174
	Baby arugula salad, 0.5 ounce	3
	Beets, 2.5 ounces	30
	Balsamic vinegar of Modena, 1 teaspoon	5
	Avocados, raw, 1.75 ounces	78
	Whole-grain mini roll	86
	Store-bought coleslaw, 1.5 ounces	132
Dinner		
Snacks		
Total		508

Optional Addition for Men: 4 ounces chenin blanc white wine (perfect with this picnic salad) = 110 calories

A Soupy Day on the Go

A day to prove you can have two fairly filling meals and a snack (or two snacks if you're male)!

MEAL	FOOD	CALORIES
Breakfast	Black coffee	0
Lunch	Leek and potato soup	120
	White bread croutons	79

MEAL	FOOD	CALORIES
Dinner	Green and White Super Soup (page 164)	76
	Chicken breast, 3.5 ounces	100
	Salsa (page 174)	14
	Broccoli, 3.5 ounces, steamed	32
	Mushrooms, 2 ounces fried with no-calorie cooking spray then heated	10
	Cream cheese with chives 1½ tablespoons	32
Snacks		
Total		463

Optional Addition for Men: 1 medium banana = 90 calories

Family-Friendly Feast

This is perfect for those days when you don't want to cook separate dishes for the family or when you don't want anyone to notice you're on a diet. Simply eat the same dishes but serve extras (granola and lots of yogurt for breakfast, extra toast with butter and cheese for lunch, portion of rice and chicken or prawns for dinner) to your family and they won't even notice.

MEAL	FOOD	CALORIES
Breakfast	Fresh raspberries	20
	Greek-style yogurt, 8 ounces	34

MEAL	FOOD	CALORIES
Lunch	Toast, 1 slice	92
	Beans, 7 ounces	144
Dinner	Mushroom Tom Yum Soup (page 163)	40
	Easy Vegetable Curry (page 159)	150
Snacks		
Total		480

Optional Addition for Men: ½ cup cooked couscous = 88 calories

Three Square (Ready-Made) Meals

Three satisfying but easily prepared meals for when you have very little time!

MEAL	FOOD	CALORIES
Breakfast	Quaker Perfect Portions Cinnamon Instant Oatmeal	160
Lunch	Campbell's Soup On the Go Chicken with Mini Noodles Soup	70
Dinner	Cafe Steamers Honey Glazed Turkey and Sweet Potatoes	250
Snacks		
Total		480

Optional Addition for Men: 1 stoneground bread roll or slice bread = 80–95 calories

The Big Breakfast

Enjoy a super-satisfying breakfast OR brunch to keep you full all day!

MEAL	FOOD	CALORIES
Breakfast	2 strips lean unsmoked back bacon	106
	2 portobello mushrooms, grilled with 1 teaspoon olive oil	45
	8 cherry tomatoes on the vine	24
	1 slice whole-grain bread	90
	1 free-range pork sausage, 86 percent pork, grilled	122
	1 free-range egg, poached	75
Lunch		
Dinner		
Snacks		502
Total		

Optional Addition for Men: 4 ounces freshly squeezed orange juice (63 calories), 3.5 ounces mixed frozen berries (30 calories), either whole or blended together as a smoothie = 103 calories

Celebration Time

If you plan it carefully, you can still go to the ball. Of course, when you're eating out, calories are approximate, but these are all safe bets!

MEAL	FOOD	CALORIES
Breakfast		
Lunch	1 portion Spicy Indian Lentil & Tomato Soup (page 162)	130
Dinner	7 cherry tomatoes	21
	7 carrot sticks	35
	4 cucumber sticks	4
	2 tablespoons hummus	23
	2 tablespoons salsa	15
	1 grilled chicken wing	55
	2 pieces nigiri salmon sushi	125
Snacks	Cava, 4 ounces	94
Total		502

Optional Addition for Men: 2 Italian breadsticks (40 calories), 1 tablespoon guacamole (25 calories), 1 mini cocktail sausage (30 calorie) = 95 calories

Blank Planning Template

Use the template on the next page to plan and then monitor your own Fast Days. Record your mood and thoughts as you progress to help you work out what's the best balance for you.

There's a downloadable, printable version of the 5:2 Diet Book Meal Planner at www.the5-2dietbook.com/freebies.

The 5:2 Diet

DATE:		
MEAL	BREAKFAST	LUNCH
FOOD		
CALORIES		
MOOD & COMMENTS		
TOTAL:		

DATE:		
MEAL	DINNER	SNACKS & DRINKS
FOOD		
CALORIES		
MOOD & COMMENTS		
TOTAL:		

📓 *Kate's 5:2 Diary Part Five*

June 2013 and Beyond

The Way to Live—Forever!

Mood: Hopeful, Expectant, Optimistic
Weight on June 5, 2013: 135 Pounds
Total Lost: 26 Pounds
BMI: 23.2
Days on Diet: 300+

My number one goal on January 1, 2012, was to get back to a healthy weight by 2013, but it was a resolution I'd failed to achieve for *years*.

And now I've done it!

I know for certain this wouldn't have happened without 5:2, and I couldn't be more thrilled.

Christmas: The goose got fat, but I didn't!

Before Christmas, I was a bit nervous about how to maintain fasting with lots of social events revolving around food. I decided to be flexible and give up trying to fast during the holiday week between Christmas and New Year. I knew I might put a little weight on but also knew it would be temporary—and so it's proved. My weight loss continued into January and beyond, and most group members report they put very little weight on during holiday periods or vacations and are as enthusiastic as ever.

Winter whirlwind

It was a whirlwind winter in other ways.

I finished the first edition of this book in November and it went on sale on Kindle at the end of the month. Within days, it was topping the UK diet chart, and then in early 2013, we published a print edition, which has become a best seller here. The most rewarding part of this journey has been the many e-mails and messages from people who are every bit as excited as I am about the potential this approach has to transform lives.

Our cozy little Facebook group now has more than 6,000 members—and the forum is a great hub for even more information, with visitors from all over the world. Not a day goes by without new stories about health improvements or inspiring photos showing brilliant weight losses members have achieved.

My original diet companions have also been reporting on their progress. Andrew and his office colleagues have incredible willpower:

> *Before Christmas, we had a box of chocolates given to us as a gift—on a diet day of course! We all speculated about scoffing the lot the next day, but guess what, none of us fancied them the next day! That indeed seems to be*

an achievement—our overall appetite for eating more than we need has diminished. Most people I speak to are intrigued and usually think I'm on a food-restricted diet until I explain more. I have to say I'm a bit of an evangelist, so I am pretty good at converting people—even some real skeptics.

Like me, Tina is loving the health effects:

I think our emotional and mental wellbeing improves a lot on less food. I feel much more positive and clear-headed if that makes sense. A bit like walking out on an early crisp cold morning and feeling really alive. :) I guess that's the sharpness you mentioned. I used to take two [kinds] of blood pressure tablets, but since losing weight my blood pressure has dropped dramatically. I only discovered it because I started getting heart palpitations and went to my doctor. He took my blood pressure, then told me to stand up. As I did he actually went "whoa!" My blood pressure dropped very low. After monitoring it and seeing how low it had become, he took me off the medication and for the first time in about twenty years, I'm medication free! My friends and family all think it's a great diet, too. In fact, both my sisters-in-law, my husband's niece, and one of my friends have joined your group because they think I look great!

And Linda has been reaping the benefits too:

My mother had her six-monthly family day just after Christmas and my nephew, who I hadn't seen for six months, commented, "Good grief Linda, where's the rest of you gone?"! My only "problem" is that having eaten low-calorie foods for most of my life it's hard to eat anything like "normal" calories on my "feasting" days, so I will often eat a couple of biscuits or have a glass of wine to make up the calories!

Scientists are busy continuing research into intermittent fasting and I'll be posting updates on www.the5-2dietbook.com, but I thought I'd end with the answers to the questions people have asked me recently.

Be honest—have you considered giving up this diet?

Not once. With pretty much every other diet I've undertaken, I've already given up by month four. On this one, I might have the odd day when circumstances change—I fancy going out to celebrate something, or a friend calls out of the blue. But there's no beating myself up. I simply switch the Fast Day to tomorrow. This isn't all or nothing—it's about a small but permanent change.

Will you abandon 5:2 once you reach the target?

No. In fact, I've already passed my target. I now feel good about my body and am looking forward to the summer. I've also started doing the "Couch to 5K" running plan. I usually fast one or two days a week, as a kind of check-in on portion size, and, of course, for the health benefits. I weigh myself regularly, because it's a good way to keep the pounds from creeping back on. Though I hope the changes to my appetite will also work in my favor there too, and I will maintain the weight loss for good this time.

Is this just another diet craze that will be forgotten by next Christmas?

My opinion—shared by many others—is that this really is different. It's not about cutting out entire food groups, or eating strange foods dreamed up by the diet industry. For me, it's about people who are overwhelmed by choice and the availability of food being helped to make better decisions. The appetite element, the flexibility, the health benefits, and the all-round sustainability of this diet make it different.

Plus, it's a "craze" that happens to have been around a very, very long time, from the unavoidable and frankly scary feast-or-famine lifestyle of early man to the instructions to fast contained in so many religions. A respite or retreat from excess is something that has worked for humanity for many centuries. In the twentieth century, those who could turn their back on the feeling of hunger did, but now I've rediscovered what appetite and food mean to me.

A Sense of Perspective

I'm writing this on the evening of a Fast Day when I've eaten only one main meal, with no hunger pangs or ill effects. It reminds me how lucky we are to be able to choose what and when we eat. Fasting has done much more than help me lose weight—it's helped me regain control over my eating habits and made me look forward to my next meal as one of the pleasures of life.

I really hope you've been inspired by the stories in this book of the fantastic dieters who shared their struggles and their successes. If you'd like your 5:2 journey to continue after this book, join us. We're @the52diet on Twitter, at facebook.com/groups/the52diet, and on the new website, www.the5-2dietbook.com, where you can join the forums, find recipes or download free tools to make life easier.

You can also get in touch with me there—I'd love to hear from you!

Finally, if you've enjoyed this book and would like to recommend it to others, I'd be so grateful if you'd think about leaving a review.

In the meantime, keep feasting, keep fasting, and keep enjoying life! Somehow, it all tastes so much better these days.

Kate x

APPENDIX

BMI Chart

	Normal						Overweight				
BMI	19	20	21	22	23	24	25	26	27	28	29
Height	Weight										
4'8"	91	96	100	105	110	115	119	124	129	134	138
4'9"	94	99	104	109	114	119	124	128	133	138	143
5'	97	102	107	112	118	123	128	133	138	143	148
5'1"	100	106	111	116	122	127	132	137	143	148	153
5'2"	104	109	115	120	126	131	136	142	147	153	158
5'3"	107	113	118	124	130	135	141	146	152	158	163
5'4"	110	116	122	128	134	140	145	151	157	163	169
5'5"	114	120	126	132	138	144	150	156	162	168	174
5'6"	118	124	130	136	142	148	155	161	167	173	179
5'7"	121	127	134	140	146	153	159	166	172	178	185
5'8"	125	131	138	144	151	158	164	171	177	184	190
5'9"	128	135	142	149	155	162	169	176	182	189	196
5'10"	132	139	146	153	160	167	174	181	188	195	202
5'11"	136	143	150	157	165	172	179	186	193	200	208
6'	140	147	154	162	169	177	184	191	199	206	213
6'1"	144	151	159	166	174	182	189	197	204	212	219
6'2"	148	155	163	171	179	186	194	202	210	218	225
6'3"	152	160	168	176	184	192	200	208	216	224	232
6'4"	156	164	172	180	189	197	205	213	221	230	238

BMI Chart

BMI	Obese										Extreme Obesity			
	30	31	32	33	34	35	36	37	38	39	40	41	42	43
Height	Weight													
4'8"	143	148	153	158	162	167	172	177	181	186	191	196	201	205
4'9"	148	153	158	163	168	173	178	183	188	193	198	203	208	212
5'	153	158	163	168	174	179	184	189	194	199	204	209	215	220
5'1"	158	164	169	174	180	185	190	195	201	206	211	217	222	227
5'2"	164	169	175	180	186	191	196	202	207	213	218	224	229	235
5'3"	169	175	180	186	191	197	203	208	214	220	225	231	237	242
5'4"	174	180	186	192	197	204	209	215	221	227	232	238	244	250
5'5"	180	186	192	198	204	210	216	222	228	234	240	246	252	258
5'6"	186	192	198	204	210	216	223	229	235	241	247	253	260	266
5'7"	191	198	204	211	217	223	230	236	242	249	255	261	268	274
5'8"	197	203	210	216	223	230	236	243	249	256	262	269	276	282
5'9"	203	209	216	223	230	236	243	250	257	263	270	277	284	291
5'10"	209	216	222	229	236	243	250	257	264	271	278	285	292	299
5'11"	215	222	229	236	243	250	257	265	272	279	286	293	301	308
6'	221	228	235	242	250	258	265	272	279	287	294	302	309	316
6'1"	227	235	242	250	257	265	272	280	288	295	302	310	318	325
6'2"	233	241	249	256	264	272	280	287	295	303	311	319	326	334
6'3"	240	248	256	264	272	279	287	295	303	311	319	327	335	343
6'4"	246	254	263	271	279	287	295	304	312	320	328	336	344	353

Resources

The links and resources here have been organized chapter by chapter, to help you discover more on the subjects that matter to you. Where a link is very long, I've used a "bit.ly" link, which is simply a way of shortening the address—just type the short link into your browser.

I've put together a free downloadable list of all the links, to make it easier to follow up Internet resources. It's available at www.the5-2dietbook.com and will save you a lot of typing! Please do bear in mind that although I've checked through these links, I can't be responsible for any outside content.

Part One: The 5:2 Revolution

The Math of Weight Loss—and Why Fasting Adds Up

Dr. John Briffa on why BMI is not the best predictor of future health: http://bit.ly/W3i2N r

The British *Daily Telegraph* on the height/weight ratio as a
  measure of CVD risk: http://bit.ly/UYneDE
Plus summary of one study: http://1.usa.gov/SwIwLe
Abstract of study on intermittent calorie restriction by
  Krista Varady: 1.usa.gov/fLnc4v
The Mark's Daily Apple website has a focus on "primal
  living" but there's a terrific amount of information
  on fasting, including summaries on the science: http://
  bit.ly/Uui9DP

The Fasting Recharge

Simple description of apoptosis http://science.howstuff
  works.com/life/cellular-microscopic/apoptosis.htm
  and autophagy http://www.news-medical.net/health/
  Autophagy-What-is-Autophagy.aspx
Summary of various studies focusing on fighting aging in
  mice: http://bit.ly/SwOFHh
News article on experiment on mice genetically
  engineered to produce more FGF21: http://bit.ly/
  V8DiDM
Plastic surgeon James Johnson carried out research on
  people with asthma undertaking his UpDayDownDay
  Diet: http://bit.ly/TUPKXF
Overview of fasting research by Krista Varady and Marc
  Hellerstein. Their review of studies was published in
  2007 so is a little out of date, but it contains a great
  summary of the diverse research: http://bit.ly/113ykL3

A more recent review http://bit.ly/ShaV4h examines more studies.

The Genesis Breast Cancer Prevention Centre in Manchester, UK, is at genesisuk.org and has run a number of studies. There's a summary of one here http://1.usa.gov/XxFkNn and download a guide to the work being done by Genesis here http://bit.ly/100sv2n

These two blogs explore whether women's physiological responses to fasting are different to men's: http://bit.ly/XxFowH and http://bit.ly/X7mTNi

The Hunger Game—Fasting is Good for the Brain

Link about BDNF, a protein with a key role in brain health: http://www.dnalc.org/view/1465-BDNF-Gene.html

Interesting pieces on the research into not only for Alzheimer's and other forms of dementia, but also strokes: http://bit.ly/V5ewTv

Fasting advocate Mark Sisson on brain function and fasting: http://bit.ly/QPanph

Part Two: 5:2 Your Way

Step One: How Much Do You Want to Lose, and How Much Can You Afford to Eat?

www.myfitnesspal.com/tools

Step Two: Your First Fast

Article on one recent survey about secretive male dieters:
   http://bit.ly/Yu9OmL
Potassium, magnesium, or calcium to reduce cramps:
   http://bit.ly/TsrDvY
Kiwi fruits and sleep disorders: http://1.usa.gov/W3jwqN
The Diabetes UK site has very clear information about GI
   values and diets as well as lots about the disease itself:
   http://bit.ly/Tv2B2Y
Science Daily has lots of interesting articles, written in
   fairly jargon-free language: start with this one http://
   bit.ly/QPeAsS and then follow the links to other pieces
   that reflect your own interests!

Step Three: Review, Revise, Revitalize

The getsomeheadspace.com site offers a free introductory
   trial of meditations as well as some really useful
   downloads, including one on mindful eating. Read
   more about mindfulness and food in the *Independent*
   http://ind.pn/QsEwJp and the *New York Times* http://
   nyti.ms/U4Fis5
UK NHS analysis of study on exercising after fasting:
   http://bit.ly/Vgv6Uh

Part Three: Eating the 5:2 Way

Food and Fasting Tips

How chiles might help with fat burning and increasing the
metabolism: http://bit.ly/11jyZHs

Breakfasts

Guide to analyzing GI and other health aspects of your
daily cereal: http://bit.ly/QPcolf

A study on the potential drawbacks of cereal bars: http://
bbc.in/U4FCXC

Read about the nutritional values of different types of
yogurt: http://bit.ly/V5hF5u

Main Meals

Scientific study on the satiating effect of soup:
http://bbc.in/YahY4T

There's lots of information about shirataki noodles
here: http://bit.ly/V5iFGS

Tangerines and the potential of nobiletin: http://bit.ly/
WFklpb

Medicinal benefits of vinegar: http://bit.ly/Ssvdcg

General Fasting and Healthy Eating Links:

The *Horizon* Eat, Fast, Live Longer program, which
inspired so many, has its own page at http://www.bbc
.co.uk/programmes/b01lxyzc: it no longer shows the
entire program, but there are some clips.

There's also an article by presenter Dr. Mosley about his
experiences on the BBC site http://bbc.in/UuhPVU

as well as a similar one in the British *Daily Telegraph* http://bit.ly/11jCMol

Recipes

The excellent BBC Good Food recipes site allows you to specify courses, ingredients, preparation time, and calorie counts—the user ratings are incredibly useful too: http://bit.ly/SsvbkI. You will need to use a conversion table or web page to change the recipes to U.S. measurements but it is worth that little effort for some fabulous dishes.

Conversions from cups to grams: http://bit.ly/U4Ft6A

Some brilliant UK bloggers are now posting images of their own recipes for 5:2 days: be inspired by lovely pictures and ideas: http://pinterest.com/LavenderLovage/5-2-diet-recipes-for-fast-days

And my own Pinterest page shows some of the dishes I've been experimenting with lately: http://pinterest.com/katewritesbooks/my-5-2-diet

Forums

Our 5:2 Diet Group on Facebook is very friendly, and anyone can see the entries: http://www.facebook.com/groups/the52diet but to post, you'll have to ask to join. There is also a new forum at the5-2dietbook.com

Appendix

The BMI chart was adapted from: http://www.nhlbi.nih.gov/guidelines/obesity/bmi_tbl.pdf

Further Reading

The Hairy Dieters: How to Love Food and Lose Weight by
Dave Myers and Si King
This recipe book gets the thumbs up from many forum
members who love the Bikers' brilliant ideas for Fast
Days.

The Fast Diet: Lose Weight, Stay Healthy, and Live Longer
with the Simple Secret of Intermittent Fasting by
Michael Mosley and Mimi Spencer
Dr. Mosley was the presenter of the *Horizon* program,
and his scientific background makes the science
impeccable, while his co-author is strong on the
practical side.

5:2 Fasting and Fitness: Easy Science in Layman's Terms by
Linda Gruchy
This is a great little e-book written by one of the
original members of my Facebook group. Linda has
a background in sports science and nutrition, and she
has a terrific writing style. This book answers many

of the questions you may have about how food and exercise affect the body.

The 2-Day Diet: Diet Two Days a Week. Eat the Mediterranean Way for Five by Michelle Harvie and Tony Howell
This book hasn't been published at the time of writing but it comes from the Genesis team in Manchester, whose work on breast cancer prevention is making a major contribution in the field, and I'm looking forward to reading it.

The Alternate-Day Diet: Turn on Your "Skinny Gene," Shed the Pounds, and Live a Longer and Healthier Life by James B. Johnson and Donald R. Laub
Johnson's book goes into a lot of detail about the science, if you want to know more. I'm not as keen on the meal plans or use of diet replacement meals, but you might be!

Index

Some Final Thanks

To Araminta, Peta, and Sophie for being there at the start of the 5:2 journey. Together, we're a lean, mean slimming machine.

To all the fabulous members of the 5:2 Diet Facebook group, and especially to the people who told me everything about their diet history, health concerns, and experiences of fasting. Thanks especially to Linda for her great graph and insights, and Jenny M. for her fantastic response to the early draft.

To Jenn and Julie Cohen and Julie Boyer for help with U.S. foods and equivalents. To Su Quinn for being so inspirational with her publishing experiences.

To Katherine and everyone at Ulysses Press for helping to make the U.S. edition a reality!

To my parents for teaching me to love food and eating out.

To Rich for making me step away from my desk occasionally to eat, sleep, and think about something other than fasting.

Special thanks to the BBC *Horizon* team for making a program that inspired so many people to try this approach to food and health.

Most of all, we all owe thanks to the many scientists who are pioneering so much incredible work in the field of fasting and health. We are hungry to see what you come up with next!

About the Author

Before becoming an acclaimed diet-book author and novelist, Kate Harrison worked as a journalist in newspapers and then at the BBC. She was a reporter and producer in news, investigative/consumer shows, food programs, and documentaries. Kate is the author of ten novels, including the Secret Shopper series, *The Boot Camp* (Orion 2012), and the teen thriller series Soul Beach. She has written about health, food, and relationships for a range of newspapers and magazines, including *Cosmopolitan*, the *Times of London*, and the *Irish Independent*. She has appeared on TV worldwide talking about *The 5:2 Diet*, which has been translated into more than a dozen languages. Visit her at www.kate-harrison.com.